About the Author

Christopher Connolly is a consultant with The Sporting Body-mind Ltd, an organisation which teaches professional and amateur athletes mental training techniques and skills for improving their body/mind co-ordination. He has worked with Tottenham Hotspur Football Club and a number of national sports associations in Britain, Europe and the USA. With a degree in Psychology, he is also trained in the Feldenkrais Method of neuromuscular integration and in Psychosynthesis. He travels widely, lecturing and giving courses, and is guest lecturer on Mental Training at the Royal Academy of Music. Christopher Connolly is co-author, with John D. Syer, of *Sporting Body, Sporting Mind*, and is also a contributor to the *Vogue Exercise Book*. He lives in London and enjoys watersports and athletics.

Hetty Einzig is a freelance journalist whose interest in health, growth and fitness – in particular in relation to women – developed while she was reading Modern Languages at Cambridge University. She believes that exercise, diet, psychology and the arts are not separate fields but interact crucially for full health and growth. Currently editor of the Mind and Body section of *Time Out*, she has also written for the *Sunday Times* magazine, *Harpers & Queen*, *Vogue* and *New Health*. In 1983, with co-author Geoffrey Cannon, she wrote the bestselling *Dieting Makes You Fat*, and she is also co-author, with Dr Norma Williams, of *The New Guide to Women's Health*.

Acknowledgements

We would like to thank all our friends and family who have supported us unfailingly through the saga that this book became. In particular, John Syer, who was always there, Trudy Barton and Schaun Tozer for the hot soup and laughter, Naomi and Dennis Milne for their love and warmth, Georgina Dobrée, unwavering in her encouragement, Susan Einzig for her concern and practical support, and Geoffrey Cannon for pushing us right at the start.

We would also like to thank Kathy Crilley, Barbara Dale, Clare Hayes, Sumi Komo, Tony Lycholat, Olga Rutherford, David Steele and all the others who helped us to get it right.

A special thank you must go to Deborah Rogers, our agent, and Gail Rebuck, our publisher, for backing what started simply as 'a good idea', to Sarah Wallace for her enthusiasm and endless supply of Perrier, and finally to Caroline Ball who more than anyone else helped us transform an Ugly Duckling of a manuscript into a Stage Two Swan.

The Fitness Jungle

Stage 2 Fitness: The Exercise Survival Guide

CHRISTOPHER CONNOLLY and HETTY EINZIG

CENTURY
LONDON   MELBOURNE   AUCKLAND   JOHANNESBURG

Published in paperback by Century Hutchinson Ltd in 1987

First published in 1986 by Century Hutchinson Ltd,
Brookmount House, 62–65 Chandos Place, Covent Garden,
London WC2N 4NW

Century Hutchinson Australia Pty Ltd,
PO Box 496, 16–22 Church Street, Hawthorn, Victoria 3122

Century Hutchinson New Zealand Ltd,
PO Box 40-086, Glenfield, Auckland 10, New Zealand

Century Hutchinson South Africa Pty Ltd,
PO Box 337, Bergvlei, 2012 South Africa

Set in Plantin by Avocet Marketing Services, Bicester
Printed in Great Britain by
St Edmundsbury Press, Bury St Edmunds, Suffolk
Bound by Butler & Tanner Ltd, Frome, Somerset

British Library Cataloguing in Publication Data

Connolly, Christopher
   The fitness jungle: stage 2 fitness:
   the exercise survival guide.
   1. Exercise   2. Physical fitness
   I. Title   II. Einzig, Hetty
   613.7'1   RA781

ISBN 0-7126-1538-5

Contents

The Fitness Jungle

Run for your Life. Work that Body. Fit not Fat. No one can remember any more who coined these and similar catch phrases, but they have become as familiar as the old maxim: an apple a day keeps the doctor away. In the space of a decade we have witnessed a social revolution: fitness has become the new morality. Individuals from all sections of society and from all walks of life have espoused the cause and mouthed its dogma. The skinny, hippy sixties gave way to the fitness-conscious seventies and on to the muscled, honed and healthy eighties. The message was enthralling, inspiring:

> The short-term excitement and intensity created by the over-blown desire to win at all costs can be replaced by a more durable excitement and intensity springing from the heart of the athletic experience itself [writes the visionary educator George Leonard in *The Ultimate Athlete*]. We may well discover that sports and physical education, reformed and refurbished, may provide us with the best possible path to personal enlightenment and social transformation in this age.

On a more pragmatic level Jane Fonda, queen of fitness, put it with persuasive personal sincerity:

> I do not claim that a strong, healthy woman is automatically going to be a progressive, decent sort of person. Obviously other factors are involved in that. But I am sure that one's innate intelligence and instinct for good can be enhanced through fitness.

Stage One Fitness – Out of Control

There is no doubt that the benefits of the fitness boom have been phenomenal. It has changed people's attitudes to health at a fundamental level. Exercise has now become an integral part of health cultivation and maintenance, both in the private home and in the business and medical spheres. This Stage One of the fitness revolution got people out of their chairs and moving.

But in the early 1980s doubts began to emerge. Distortion and dissension were rife. The numbers of joggers and aerobics devotees were still growing and a 1985 publicity blurb for one sports shoe chain enthused: 'Woman and man were made to run. And what was once a prerequisite for survival has become a passport to health and fitness.' But reports of sports injuries increased, deaths during exercise hit the headlines. In his book *The Exercise Myth*, Dr Henry Solomon, an American cardiologist, wrote:

> If the worst thing that could be said about exercise is that it doesn't prevent coronary heart disease or death, then those who enjoy the sweat and pain would have no reason not to 'go for it' . . . But people don't just die in spite of exercise. They die because of it.

Such contradictions highlight the confusion resulting from the uninformed and gung-ho attitudes that characterized Stage One of the fitness boom.

It was in this climate of confusion and heated disagreement that the idea for this book came about. We found ourselves in the middle of a fitness jungle: health and fitness had become priorities in many people's lives but they didn't know which way to turn. Scientists and physiologists, epidemiologists and cardiologists with their electromyographs, stress tests, specialized jargon and statistics; pronouncements on chic, flair, style and trends from the seducers of the fashion and leisure industries; gurus and opportunists, the star, the doctor and the businessman, made up an increasingly luxuriant scene. Already by the spring of 1984 the fitness jungle had become a dangerous place for the rest of us. Claims and counter-claims as to the benefits of exercise or what sort of exercise was suitable were filling the pages of the press and soon the bookshops too. There were accusations of narcissism and exhortations to save your body and soul and get physical. Did exercise make you live younger and longer, or kill you off?

How had these seemingly irreconcilable points of view come about to create such a jungle for us?

The fitness boom

Today's idea of fitness grew up in America during the 1950s and 60s. Between 1948 and 1958 American car ownership increased from 30 million to 67 million. Television, along with a range of labour saving devices, entered the homes of a newly prosperous American public. Activity levels, not surprisingly, went down. Tests by the American Association of Health, Physical Education and Recreation confirmed the low level of fitness in children between ten and seventeen years of age. But things began to get serious when, in 1959, in order to recruit an additional 196,000 men to meet the Berlin Crisis, the US government found that out of every seven men called up, three were rejected on physical grounds.

Amongst the general public, deaths and debilitation from heart disease were rising to epidemic proportions. The sharp increase among younger men, between 25 and 44 years of age, was particularly disturbing. Meanwhile the cost of health care was rising at the same alarming rate – in the USA from $12 billion to $70 billion between 1950 and 1970.

During the 1950s and 60s studies started to emerge showing the links between physical activity and a lower incidence of heart disease: the ground was being laid for the first stage in the fitness revolution. But the notion of fitness was still obscure, gyms were unattractive places, sports were for jocks, and the country clubs catered for the genteel round of golf and a social drink rather than for the health-conscious person.

A number of key events and social shifts from the later 1960s onwards gradually brought the voices of the scientists and epidemiologists to the public's attention.

In 1968 Dr Kenneth Cooper's book, *Aerobics*, introduced to the public the idea and the feasibility of incorporating vigorous exercise into one's lifestyle as a method of preventative health care. His conclusion was that aerobic exercise was a major key in preventing heart disease. The book, and subsequent ones by

Cooper, inspired a nation: for the first time someone was offering a clear-cut practical answer to the number one killer, and also managing to convey physiological concepts in a simple way. Throughout the 1970s people took to the streets, pools and dance studios to follow his prescription. He was effective in getting America on the move partly because the time was ripe but also because his books carried the authority of his many years of research on the value of aerobic exercise with the US Air Force. Thousands passed through his laboratory and followed his exercise regime.

Cooper's was not, of course, the only voice purveying the exercise message, but it would be another decade before there was wide-scale acceptance of just how generally destructive our sedentary lifestyles had become. As Cooper himself points out, advances in preventative health care were seen as possible only when spending on medical treatment approached that on defence. The US government panicked and pumped funds into research and ventures like Cooper's, under the auspices of the President's Council on Physical Fitness, set up by John F. Kennedy.

The second important social trend that helped fire Stage One of the fitness boom was the growth of the women's movement, with its emphasis on the rediscovery and reclaiming of female power, both political and physical. In the struggle to abolish the fragile, take-care-of-me image of femininity, women's immediate and increasing involvement in the cult of physical fitness has proved an important asset. Through running, dance, aerobics and self-defence classes, women who would not dream of describing themselves as feminists began to experience at first hand the satisfaction of feeling strong, of achieving goals, of competition, of camaraderie and the sheer sweat-n-guts of physical exertion.

The very real advance that this new-found physical prowess represents for women has been blurred by the inevitable exploitation of the trend by the media and fashion industry. It has been all too easy to focus instead on the time-honoured perspective: woman as a beautiful object to be admired, desired, joked about and used as the best-ever sales prop. From being skinny à la Twiggy, she was now 'coming on strong', as the cover of *Time* magazine put it in 1982. Jane Fonda exemplified this Catch 22 situation. The message she put forth in her

Workout book was inspiring to millions of women but at the same time the image of her honed, lean, sexy body caught many in the usual trap of aiming for a prescribed standard, a look rather than an experience – epitomized by the bronzed, muscled beauties of America's West Coast, where for many fitness has increasingly become nothing more than another posture.

The third factor in the resurgence of the body is the rise of sport as a money-spinner – and not just for the top professional athlete. While participant sport has always been a pastime, and spectator sport a popular leisure pursuit, it is only with the tremendous coverage (which increases yearly) given to it by the media, and in particular television, that sport has been brought to the forefront of people's consciousness all over the world. Sport is now a world of mega-bucks. For the 1988 Olympics the television rights alone are costing $300 million. Advertising and promotion play their part in ensuring that sporting stars and products are constantly current references. The amount of money now available for sports sponsorship has made it possible for more adolescents and young adults to pursue excellence in their sport, and the rewards to be won on the circuit in golf, tennis, skiing and a host of other sports, make it a highly attractive career. Champions have been promoted into the lime-light previously occupied by entertainment stars or politicians. Through television we have gained a more intimate relationship with these cult figures than ever before, and public adulation and emulation have increased in equal measure. The appeal to our fantasies of these young, athletic, golden and attractive stars is easy to understand.

Sporting accomplishments are becoming more than append-ages to one's curriculum vitae. Sport is no longer seen as simple recreation, it has become mainstream, and the sporting elite are taking their place alongside businessmen, intellectuals, artists and politicians as honoured professionals and respected rep-resentatives of nation, culture, race and sex.

Nor is this phenomenon limited to sport. Bruce Lee, though he may be criticized by the purists, was able to sweep past boundaries of culture and comprehension by presenting martial arts in a way that captured the imagination of tens of millions of young people.

The fitness industry has capitalized on our yearning to be like these shining heroes and heroines with the message: *you too* can go out and do it, *you can* become like this (while carefully underplaying the draconian training regimes and highly restricted lives professional sportspeople lead in order to attain their level of excellence).

These, then, are some of the factors that have combined to bring about Stage One fitness. And, in keeping with the uncontrolled growth process endemic in our age, and our belief in simple solutions, things soon got out of hand. Exercise, particularly aerobic exercise, came to be seen as a cure-all, the panacea for all ills. The pursuit of physical activity became for many an obsession.

There is in all obsessions a note of desperation, and desperation breeds imbalance. Claims, inflated by the media and a now greedy fitness industry, exceeded current physiological and epidemiological knowledge and the public came to believe that running and other strenuous exercise conferred immunity from heart disease, promised longevity, a slender, healthy youth and a fat-free, wrinkle-free and therefore trouble-free middle and old age.

In those first glory days of the fitness boom the message was simple: get out there and run, jump, hop and dance your way to perfect health and a long life. Cardiovascular fitness was the be-all and end-all and, above all, the solution to the heart disease epidemic. Fitness was equated with health, and millions in the United States and Europe gave up the drugs and got moving instead.

That equation – of fitness with health – lies at the very root of the subsequent confusion and misunderstandings which have plagued the exerciser and given rise to the spate of scare stories in the press about injuries and deaths due to exercise.

Is Fitness Bad for Your Health?

Fitness is *not* health. The term 'fitness', as it is now used, merely refers to the cardiovascular and respiratory system. To be fit means you have a strong, hard-working heart and lungs. It does *not* mean that they are free of disease, abnormalities or clogged arteries, or that the rest of your body is likewise immune to sickness. The equation of fitness with health rooted itself in the minds of male runners who came to believe that a hard-working heart must be immune to attacks and that fitness could hold at bay or even reverse the process of atherosclerosis. In aerobic dance classes, young women – the predominant participants – pounded away to the disco beat, seduced by the sci-speak of cardiovascular training, pulse taking, and 'aerobics points', while still remaining oblivious to the complexity of the fitness – health relationship.

The injuries began to mount up. The first citizen running deaths occurred. Long before the research studies into this area began to be made public the press leapt at the potential. From late 1982 the headlines started to appear: EXERCISE TEACHERS BLAMED FOR INJURIES TO YOUNG WOMEN; EXERCISE CAN SERIOUSLY DAMAGE YOUR HEALTH; FITNESS EXPERTS CAUSING DEATHS, SAYS SCIENTIST and so on. The scare was on. Hype and counter-hype, assertion and denial, protestation and recriminations started to sour the exercise field, putting off many potential exercisers and worrying those already at it.

The two main areas of concern to exercisers are injuries to the musculo-skeletal system (with also some lesser concern over hormone imbalances caused by vigorous exercise) and, secondly, the relation of cardiovascular fitness to cardiovascular disease – that is, what role does exercise have to play in staving off the heart attack? And, more urgently, will exercise actually kill me?

In the studio

A lot of media attention has focused on the high number of injuries sustained by young women in aerobic exercise classes. Studies have been difficult to undertake partly because of the lack of a clear definition as to what constitutes an aerobic exercise class and partly because of the easy-come-easy-go nature of participation in classes, hence a lack of a steady population with known health histories to monitor over a substantial period.

In Britain, physiotherapist Ruth Doodson looked at the scale of injuries among women aged 16-54 in exercise to music classes and based her conclusions on reports from 83 hospitals, private practices and sports medicine specialists in England between

March and July 1984. In total 1646 injuries were reported and the largest number of these, 648 – more than a third of the total – were to the lower back and lumbar spine. Next came Achilles tendon and lower leg injuries: 234, followed by 206 knee injuries.

Despite the sense of outrage and obvious bias that colours her report, Ms Doodson's findings are useful in their indication of the extent of the problem and in alerting the individual to the areas of the body particularly vulnerable during exercise.

In the United States the principal anti-injury champions, Drs Peter and Lorna Francis, founded the National Injury Prevention Foundation in San Diego, and in March 1983 undertook a survey of 135 instructors in the aerobic dance field. They found that over 76 per cent of them had sustained or aggravated one or more injuries from aerobic dancing, and a full 64 per cent of these were new injuries. Unlike Ms Doodson the Francises found that, for both instructors and students, the shin was the commonest site of injury, followed by the foot, back, ankle and knee, in that order. They found the major cause to be inadequate footwear and the shock impact from repeated jumping on non-resilient surfaces. The Francis study highlighted a major cause of concern: 65 per cent of the teachers were *self-taught* and only 27 per cent had attended some form of training course.

Exercise teachers have been as alarmed at this state of affairs as the general public, and, first in the United States and then in Britain, organizations were hurriedly set up in an attempt to set and supervise methods and standards (see Body Conditioning Methods, page 187).

On the track

On the track and in the park the injuries have also mounted up. A number of surveys indicate that it is the knees of joggers and runners that are most at risk, accounting for around 40-50 per cent of all running injuries, with lower leg injuries a distant second. In a paper, 'The Most Common Problems Seen in a Metropolitan Sports Injury Clinic' (reported in *The Physician and Sports Medicine*), running/jogging came top of the league table, accounting for 32.6 per cent of the injuries seen by a New

York clinic, with basketball, the second, well behind with 9.7 per cent of injuries. Almost 76 per cent of all injuries occurred during recreational sport (as opposed to 15.1 per cent during school-related activities) and men visiting the clinic outnumbered women by two to one.

But perhaps even more significant is the evidence from another American study, by Clement *et al*, which showed that while 60 per cent of the patients visiting a sports physician were men, it was women under the age of 30 who ran the greatest *risk* of overuse injuries due to physical predisposition. And other researchers have confirmed this finding. While women tend to be more flexible, thereby incurring fewer muscle strains or tears than men, their skeletal characteristics land them in trouble in other areas. Wider pelvises and the resultant inward angle of their thigh bones can lead to chronic knee conditions. In addition, their curved calf bones are less efficient at absorbing the impact of the foot hitting the ground or studio floor and consequently are more susceptible to stress fractures. These findings are increasingly causing some people to question whether, in the end, running is a suitable sport for the female exerciser, for no amount of well-cushioned footwear or compensating running style can change anatomy. However, the 2:1 ratio of male/female patients at the above-mentioned New York clinic indicates that anatomy is not everything. Perhaps the macho approach causes more self-injury than the shape of a hip?

The mention of the suitability of strenuous exercise is also guaranteed to cause a ripple of concern among women. Until relatively recently, women were prohibited from exerting themselves, ostensibly for fear they might damage their 'delicate gynaecological plumbing' or for what the exercise might 'do' to their womanhood. Cessation of periods (amennorhea) has often been held up as evidence of the 'danger' to women of strenuous exercise, and a recent study from California also notes a diminution of oestrogen production and ovulation. The same study reports that reduced testosterone levels are found in some male exercisers; this lowers sex drive but does not affect fertility. Both the men and women in this study were running over 25 miles per week. However, an Australian study, carried out at the Gavin Institute in Sydney, found that in men the output of testosterone is *increased* when athletes participate in energetic swimming or rowing events, and higher levels of blood testosterone were found even in non-athletic students who pedalled on a stationary bicycle.

The subjective response from most surveys into this area tends to be that, up to a point, exercise improves sex life. Heavy training is bound to affect the chemical balance of the body – it is being put under severe stress. With this extra stress load to contend with the body will sensibly reduce to a minimum all other claims on its energy resources. Sexual activity and reproduction require not only reserves of energy to function properly but also, particularly for conception, a stable environment. During times of high stress – physical, mental or emotional – the healthy body will usually protect itself by putting these drives into hibernation until such time as the external demands for survival are over, or reduced. Studies conducted at several Olympic games showed not only that women won medals at all times during their menstrual cycle, and that neither amennorhea nor normal menstrual flow was a major factor in performance, but also that temporary amennorhea did not affect fertility in the long term. Once heavy training ceases the body soon returns to normal.

There is no way around the fact that just as changes in internal body milieu – hormone changes, changes in heart function and so on – are bound to happen with regular, vigorous exercise (the body adapts, after all, to the demands made on it), so musculo-skeletal injury during heavy training is, to a greater or lesser extent, par for the course. Every professional athlete or dancer will confirm this. If you drive a car you are statistically more likely to have a car accident than if you don't; if you drive it five days a week the odds will be greater, and if you drive fast as well, greater still. The same goes for exercise and your body. It must be emphasized that the steep rise in the injury rate in recreational exercise over the past decade is *primarily due quite simply* to the huge numbers now exercising compared with 15 years ago.

There are four main areas or situations where injury during exercise becomes more likely. If you become aware of these and of the state of your own body then you are in a good position to take the necessary precautions.

1   Those sports which are inherently dangerous – boxing, the aggressive martial arts (judo, karate, kung fu), downhill skiing, mountain climbing, and so on.

2 Situations or activities where carelessness, poor teaching,
   poor equipment, ignorance or mass fervour may combine
   with high intensity exercise – running, aerobic exercise,
   dance, gymnastics, skiing, etc.
3 If you are starting something new. Even an experienced
   athlete, taking up aerobic dance for example, will need time
   to learn the movements, the rules, the hows and the wherefores of this new exercise form. During this learning,
   transitional period a wrong movement is highly likely, and a
   step out of place may result in a twist or knock. Statistically
   the majority of injuries happen either to the raw beginner,
   whose body is probably stiff and unyielding, or to the top
   athlete constantly pushing past his own body's limit and the
   records set by others.
4 If you are under a lot of stress in the rest of your life then any
   exercise may be adding extra strain or working against tense
   muscles, and self-destructive emotions.

The way to avoid injury is to cultivate not only awareness of
the situation and of your own state of being but also a sense of
balance. Stage One fitness has encouraged a go-for-it attitude
inherent in the Western approach to most things, and has
capitalized on many of the most self-punitive and self-destructive
traits in the puritan character: pain is good for you; competitiveness at all costs; and exercise-to-exhaustion is the road to a
beautiful body and a high score on the moral scale.

The same attitudes, with a focus more on health than beauty,
lie behind the casualties in the race against heart disease.

The heart of the matter

On 20 July 1984 the American running guru James Fixx went
out for his daily ten-mile run and half way along his route in
rural Vermont dropped dead of a heart attack. This death, like
that of 43-year-old Paul Lander, the popular, vital, exercising,
Attorney-General of New South Wales, caused many to catch
their breath and turn pale. Fixx's death had the effect of fanning
the flames of an already smouldering debate amongst the experts,
as to the effect of exercise on coronary heart disease: whether
exercise, particularly running, has a preventative effect, does no

good at all, or is positively harmful. The general public was simply scared and bewildered.

Deaths during exercise are, in fact, rare. Coronary heart disease (CHD), on the other hand, affects, or will affect, something approaching 50 per cent of the male population in Britain by the time they reach middle age. Since the late 1960s, running and other aerobic exercise has been consistently promoted as one measure in the fight to combat this epidemic: since one of the risk factors of CHD is a sedentary lifestyle, then exercise should be encouraged. It was a small leap for the collective imagination – encouraged by writers like Fixx – to see running as the universal panacea, providing a golden cloak of invulnerability against this number one killer.

Jim Fixx was a victim of this dangerously simplistic belief. At the age of 36 he was a man headed for a heart attack: he smoked two packets of cigarettes a day and was overweight. His family history was against him: his father had had a heart attack at only 35 and died eight years later. He began running to regain fitness, stopped smoking, lost 50 lb and became an ardent competitive runner and marathoner. But even though Fixx was in a high CHD risk category he still refused to go for regular checks and stress tests. His autopsy revealed severe coronary artery disease with some of his arteries 90 per cent clogged up.

It is probable that before Fixx began to run regularly the atherosclerotic process was already well under way and that his running and lifestyle changes slowed the progression of the disease. Cardiovascular training encourages the growth of the coronary collateral vessel network (that is, the subsidiary capillaries supplying the heart) which takes over from the furred up and dying arteries. This enables those with CHD to function normally, even very well, despite sometimes advanced atherosclerosis. At the time of his death, for instance, Fixx was running 80 miles a week. But neither many years of running nor high levels of performance provide immunity against cardiac events. According to Dr Steven van Camp, cardiologist at San Diego University, had Fixx not subscribed so to the hero image and undergone regular exercise stress tests he might have undertaken bypass surgery (which today carries only a 1 per cent mortality rate) and would probably still be alive today. But Dr Henry Solomon, a New York cardiologist, does not agree with the value of stress tests. He contends that they are relatively insensitive and crude, and cannot determine the *stage* of CHD in the patient. They are also costly and not widely available, certainly in Britain.

More important perhaps, than stress tests, is to encourage those who know they are at risk to watch out for what the cardiologists term 'prodromal' symptoms. The medical definition is: any changes from usual health considered important by the individual. But more specifically they refer to such signs as easy fatigability, chest pain, indigestion, or dyspnea (difficulty with breathing). These are not symptoms to be ignored or fought through. So many cardiac victims are alexithymic, that is 'colourblind' to exhaustion and the damaging effects of high arousal on a tired body. In these cases the 'he-man syndrome' can lead to death. If the individual cares sufficiently to listen to his own body and take heed of the messages it is giving him then a heart attack may be averted.

In the key Rhode Island survey of the families of those who had died during recreational exercise, conducted by Professor Paul Thompson and colleagues, 79 per cent of respondants to the questionnaire noted prodromal symptoms shortly before death, but the victims chose to ignore them. Clearly a change in awareness of, and attitude to, CHD is called for.

Rhode Island provided a unique opportunity to study a stable population of unselected individuals – hence the importance of the findings. The study focused on the deaths during recreational exercise of 81 people in the state of Rhode Island between January 1975 to May 1982. Of the 81 deaths only one was a woman. The majority of the deaths occurred during or within seconds of exertion and in 88 per cent of the cases death was presumed to be due to atherosclerotic heart disease (which, as in James Fixx's case, builds up over many years and is not abolished by exercise). Golf, jogging and swimming, in that order, were associated with over half the deaths. But remember that the age range of golfers is generally higher than for other sports; in Thompson's sample the mean age of the golfers was 59, and of the joggers, 48. Most of the deaths occurred in the 50–60 age group. Of the few deaths that occurred in the below 30 age range two were due to congenital cardiovascular disease. This tends to be the main cause of death in exercisers under 30 – although the risk is tiny and deaths very rare.

The authors conclude that while they cannot calculate the

incidence of death during exercise or its risk compared to other activities (due to the unavailability of data on time spent exercising), *they see the risk of death during exercise as very small.*

Most cardiac arrests are triggered by sudden, straining movement and this could as likely be during sex, on the toilet, dashing for a bus, or lifting a heavy suitcase, as during exercise. Because of its focus, Thompson's study is usually interpreted by the anti-exercise lobby as supporting their claims, but Thompson himself draws different conclusions from his results. 'If you were to ask me what is the safest way to spend the next *hour*,' he commented, 'then I would say: sit down and relax. But sitting down is probably the most dangerous way to spend your *whole life*. The benefits of a lifetime of physical activity far outweigh any risks of exercise.'

Dr Peter Nixon, consultant cardiologist at the Charing Cross Hospital, London, would agree. Nixon's cardiac unit is one of the more advanced in Britain. Whereas bed rest is still the principal treatment for most cardiac patients in Britain, Nixon gets his patients moving, gently, only after they have had sufficient rest to recover from the rigours of the attack or operation, and when they can be trusted not to re-exhaust themselves with too much effort. But his approach differs crucially from the standard exercise-is-best attitude of many cardiologists today. Nixon has devised what he calls *The Human Function Curve* which charts the course of an individual in relationship to performance and arousal. The upward slope is one of healthy tension, ability to cope with stress, enjoyment of life, exercise and activity. At the apex is 'healthy fatigue'. If we allow ourselves to go on being aroused, or attempting to perform or fulfil

The Human Function Curve

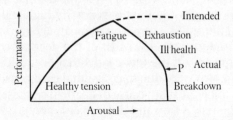

P = the point at which even minimal arousal may precipitate a breakdown

our duties *beyond* this point without taking rest, then we start on the downslope of exhaustion. This downslope becomes, more accurately, a spiral: we try harder to fight the exhaustion, become more debilitated, slip further down, try even harder and so on. Our attempt to close the gap between what we can actually do and what we think is expected of us only widens it. High stress levels interfere with the restorative value of sleep and so the situation is aggravated further – a typical description of someone headed for a heart attack.

The Human Function Curve offers a guide to self-help and to those training or prescribing exercise regimes for the middle-aged. Nixon summarizes his views on the role of exercise in coronary heart disease:

> Exercise is desirable when people are on the upslope of the Human Function Curve, in an anabolic mode. The same exercise can be applied fruitlessly, cause illness or precipitate a breakdown according to the patient's position on the downslope. It is therefore essential for a trainer to be able to judge his client's position. Many trainers come from the athletic field and do not appreciate the frequent existence of a downslope mode, and proximity to catastrophe, of people who volunteer for exercise programmes in middle age. Young athletes can be stretched to 100 per cent performance, but the middle-aged unfit must be watched for several months before they go beyond 60-75 per cent of maximum.

The bulk of the evidence that has accumulated over the past 40 years of study says that exercise has an important role to play in the prevention or alleviation of cardiovascular disease. How, or why, or how much, we do not yet know. What we *do* know is that sedentary is not better, associated as it is with all the ills of a Western lifestyle: poor circulation, poor digestion, constipation and other intestinal disorders, stiffness, back problems, obesity, depression, fatigue, low level chronic anxiety, and the more serious such as some cancers, arthritis, diabetes, osteoporosis and coronary heart disease.

It is still early days. The general public – as opposed to athletes – have only been exercising with intensity and in large numbers for a relatively short period, about fifteen years at the outside, and have been studied for even less. The first researches into injuries, exercise-related deaths, the relation of fitness to health and the role of cardiovascular fitness in heart disease are only now emerging and must be taken for what they are: investigations into the *current* situation. They are not the last word, and recommendations made by experts are just that – recommendations, not rules to be followed blindly.

Stage Two Fitness – A Sense of Balance

Respected voices among the experts are now speaking up against the fanaticism in the fitness scene and even contradicting their own earlier recommendations.

The epidemiologist Ralph Paffenbarger for years advocated strenuous physical activity as a possible safeguard against heart disease. He found that expenditure of energy of 2000 calories or more per week above that needed for daily living seemed to provide protection from CHD. The exercise enthusiasts interpreted this to mean that 20 miles of running per week (the equivalent needed to burn 2000 calories) was essential for cardiovascular health.

Now Paffenbarger and others are stating that it is likely that less vigorous exercise, such as walking or tennis, and exercise for shorter periods of time, offer a decreased risk of heart disease and will contribute to fitness. Epidemiologist Ronald Laporte says that only five to eight miles of running per week in addition to normal daily activities would probably bring the total of calories expended up to the magic 2000 calories per week mark.

As the studies are increasingly showing, taking up a vigorous exercise regime – all gung-ho and hearts-apounding – is not the simple answer. The balance between fitness and health is a delicate one. To remain in good health the body protects the homeostasis (balance) of its internal milieu by giving us clear messages: thirst prevents dehydration, fatigue prevents exhaustion, aches and pains help prevent more serious damage. But in the same way that we can learn intellectual concepts or change our personalities so our bodies can change and adapt to new demands: our metabolism slows down and we store fat in times of famine; our pulse rate, adrenalin secretion and muscle responses are heightened in times of stress and danger, and over the long-term extra demand on the heart if properly graded, will make the heart muscle grow stronger and more efficient. Health is a constant shifting balance between homeostasis and adaptation.

Many people today live in almost constant states of arousal, experiencing anxiety, demands, excitement or fear, anger or depression in quick succession. In this situation, exercise, which is a recognized and measurable physical stress on the body, may not be the refreshing release from tension or the training for the heart and lungs it is thought to be. It may be a huge additional strain on an already over-stressed body, and even in some cases, the final straw that tips the individual into breakdowns, illness, severe injury or heart attack. For true health the role of exercise is to enhance the body's ability to adapt and then return to homeostasis, the state of calm and balance where the body systems, including the immune defences against illness, can function at their best.

The 'downslope' described by Dr Nixon is a subtle thing. You may feel highly active and stimulated and yet be already slipping quietly down towards exhaustion. It is not just a question of being over-tired or of doing too much; you may be over-socializing, not sleeping well enough, using too much will-power to complete your tasks or you may be falling into the dangerous trap of seeing yourself as invulnerable, indispensable, infallible, or even immortal. We talk of people in this state as living off 'nervous energy'. Attitudes, awareness, environment, our friends and support system and much more, all play a part in our health. And our ability to recognize those downslope periods and adapt, learning to say no, for instance, or altering our expectations of ourselves, are essential for recovery of homeostasis and health. They are two of the principal new skills necessary for the next stage of fitness: self-awareness and self-regulation. So the notion that a certain fixed amount of exercise is right for everyone, or even that one regime can be tailored to the individual, is too crude. What is the right amount for one person's lifestyle may be a heavy load for another's, and what feels right for you this week may be one run or swim too many the next.

The lack of balance manifested in Stage One of the exercise boom saw aerobic fitness promoted to the exclusion of other forms of fitness training and saw the levels of exercise stepped up and up – from the weekly keep-fit class to nightly aerobics, from a 20-minute run three times a week to 40 or 60 hours a week or 80 miles on the road and a marathon twice yearly. It is hard to shake the more-must-be-better attitude that lies behind the very fabric of our culture.

In contrast to the Western idea of exercising to exhaustion, the Chinese make the analogy with saving money: the idea is not to continuously expend energy but to build up capital and only spend the interest. This is the way, say the sages, to a long and healthy life: less show, more building up of inner strength.

Paradigms and paradoxes

The mass movement towards incorporating physical exercise within a more active lifestyle is really a reflection of a much more fundamental concern for the whole of our bodies: what we eat, how we dress, how we move, when we work, how we relax and how we generally use and abuse ourselves throughout our life.

There is a growing acceptance of the truth that health in its widest sense begins at home, and must rest in our own hands. This shift, still far from complete, constitutes the fourth factor in the growth of the fitness boom. It is the one which, because it reaches deeper, more basic needs, and confronts central issues in contemporary society, has made the fitness revolution an enduring trend instead of a passing fad – and has been the impetus behind this book.

But the thing which confuses believers and critics alike is that the outward manifestation of the fitness scene actually runs counter to the motivations that have sparked the mass move-ment at the grass roots level. The one is typical of the unruly growth process and excesses of our age, the other is an integral part of the reassertion of some basic truths, and is linked to the need to relate to ourselves and to the world around us in a conscious, stable and controlled way. *But what a paradox!* The more we try to gain control of ourselves the more we are swept up in a mass movement run amok.

The world of sports and fitness activities has experienced nothing so much as a nuclear explosion: uncontrolled expansion at a furious pace, with excessive energy, distortions and loss of individual control. It is as if our assertive energy – our drive to explore, conquer, understand and create – which is the essence of our humanity, has taken on a furious momentum of its own. In a world where overload is the norm, where values and purpose change overnight, where fragmentation is rife, there has come to be little room for a sense of control over our lives and ourselves.

The pathological expressions of the profound anxiety caused by this state of affairs are numerous. One of them is the desperate need, felt initially by women and now by men too, to control our bodies. We diet them, starve them, feed them with supplements and high protein diets. We exercise and pummel them to make them slim and fit, strong and lean. We counter the ravages of age with plastic surgery or sophisticate the face of youth with make-up and high fashion.

We cultivate and display our sexual promise and yet with the outbreak of first herpes and then AIDS, promiscuous sexual contact is fraught with fear and mistrust. Cancer still remains unremittent and rife. It seems that the hundreds of millions of pounds invested in research lead always nearer to some imminent revelation: the final cancer cure. Yet promise after promise succeeds only in defining the problem without providing the answer.

But from the midst of these paradoxes there do seem to be some new models or paradigms emerging, some new means of organizing our experience in a way which allows us to escape the escalation of explosive growth and regain some inner sense of balance and direction.

In the field of medicine, the inability of the National Health Service and high-tech medicine to cope with a chronically unwell society has been exposed from within and without. While man has at last walked on the moon and heart transplants have become a reality, the so-called diseases of civilization – heart disease, diabetes, cancer, stomach and gut disorders, arthritis and psychological disorders, to name a few of the major ones – have risen to epidemic proportions in the West, and for all its superb technological achievement neither the social nor the medical institutions have been able to stem the tide. But meanwhile self-help organizations, alternative therapies, preventive and health cultivation methods, nutrition, relaxation, meditation, massage and other simple tools for well being have emerged and are rapidly being accepted.

On another level, politics has seen the emergence of movements such as CND and the ecology parties as political forces rather than powerless protestors, in answer to the increasing frustration felt by ordinary people at the infighting and catastrophic impulses of the 'big powers'.

In the fitness revolution this impulse has emerged as a desire to regain a sense of control over our bodies and lives from within ourselves. Not only do we want to create change but we want to know how to do it for ourselves.

The concept is an exhilarating one. Instead of feeling a victim of a vast and imponderable system run by experts, you suddenly realize that *you* are the expert on your own body, and you can make choices as to how you want to live with it. This was contributory to Cooper's success with his aerobics points system: he put the control back into the hands of the individual who, by calculating a number of factors, could organize his own training programme and regain his health. The interconnection between fitness and other health-conscious systems is becoming widespread. Running magazines now carry regular articles on the importance of nutrition and different diets; osteopaths and acupuncturists now work in training clubs and studios where once only a physiotherapist would preside. Sports psychologists, like the Sporting Bodymind team, work with athletes and teams to improve their awareness and performance. Moshe Feldenkrais, creator of a movement re-education method of the same name, began as a karate black belt and soccer player, and helped train members of the Israeli Olympic team. Martina Navratilova and Ivan Lendl atttribute their success to their dietary regimes. The tell-all stories of the stars are now full of references to macrobiotic eating and meditation, to alternative therapies, to workouts, running schedules and yoga practice.

This swing towards active participation rather than passive acceptance, towards doing rather than looking on is far more profound than a mere fashion. It is reconnecting individuals with their initial motivation for pursuing any of the health-enhancing systems emerging these days, not the least the exercise, sport, martial arts and dance systems examined in the second half of this book. Holism, and all the word implies, has become, like 'Small is Beautiful', a catchword for a change in consciousness in which the individual experiences an active part in the process of living.

Stage Two fitness

This same holistic relationship with one's body is a core concept for the next phase of the fitness revolution: Stage Two fitness. It indicates a move on from the dreams that fired Stage One to new levels: from dominating one's body to working together with the body *and* mind as a whole, to being a caretaker of one's physical well being, trusting in one's inner sense of what is right for oneself based on informed thinking and sound intuition: from dominance to dominion.

In the reassessment of such simple precepts as *mens sana in corpore sano*, or 'you have to love and respect yourself to love others', we are seeing an attempt to marry the best of high technology and scientific expertise with an acknowledgement of the validity of subjective experience, personal intuition and human common sense. A respect, in other words, for the life, growth, and experience of the individual in relationship with others.

The return to such fundamental healing arts as massage, the laying-on of hands, or simple movement forms, and the growing desire for simpler forms of eating, such as choosing foods which are lower down the food chain and unadulterated by chemicals, does not imply a total repudiation of technology. We are not seeing a repeat of the back-to-the-earth movement of the 1960s, nor the 'Me' decade of the 1970s.

As we become more aware of our bodies and the language they speak, the short-term goals of exercise most common to Stage One fitness – cardiovascular health, longevity, obesity control – have become less urgent. As the mind quietens and the panic clears people are getting in touch with deeper needs, deeper goals, more profound satisfactions. This does not invalidate those straightforward goals, it merely puts them in perspective. For example, the mechanistic approach characteristic of Stage One fitness which saw the heart simply as a pump to be trained like any other muscle to serve us more efficiently, now appears grossly simplistic and crude.

'It's so obvious,' says cardiologist Peter Nixon, 'but people constantly ignore how much the heart is connected to the emotions. You can't just perform sophisticated plumbing, you have to treat the whole person.' In the same way concentrated endurance training may improve the strength of the pump but only attention paid to the mind, hormones, tissues and other muscles, nerves and joints, to the whole person and *all* the factors affecting it, from diet to environment, relationships to work – will make for a *healthy* heart.

Stage Two fitness, now emergent, will be characterized by this greater awareness of inter-relationship. It will involve a commitment to self-knowledge and will be more concerned with self-actualization and cultivating the mind–body whole in relation to a greater whole, than with the development of sleek thighs or pulsing muscles. Well being has already taken on a wider meaning, a meaning that does not deny the pleasure in feeling beautiful, nor the satisfaction of well coordinated muscles, of a strong, effective body. Stage Two fitness does not denounce competition, strict training schedules, the single minded pursuit of success, but it *does* put them into a wider context.

When talking to people who exercise regularly about their motivations and what their activity fulfils for them, or when reading the comments of professional sportspeople or the evidence of the experts, certain themes recur regularly. In the next chapter, Personal Goals, we have identified these and organized them into seven broad categories. In this way, when it comes to choosing the right movement form for yourself, you will be able better to identify your own motivations, or find confirmation of your secret hopes and expectations, or indeed, re-inforcement of your own experiences.

To get through any jungle one needs knowledge of the terrain, understanding of its laws, the right equipment and support, and finally a real sense that we do have a *choice* in our journey – to go this way or that, pursue this exercise form or that, try this route and change one's mind, forge ahead or rest a while. The chapter entitled Know Your Body is an attempt to distil the prodigious amount of physiological and anatomical research conducted over the years on the body into a brief overview of the three basic systems within the body which are all directly involved in the organization and performance of movement. An active involvement in Stage Two fitness on your part requires some basic knowledge of the inner workings of your body. This is the map of the territory. Use it as you would use any map: to consult when you don't recognize the terrain.

The chapter on Physical Goals will help to show how different approaches to training will produce different physiological developments in your body. You need to know what your physical goals are and the proper training approach to them.

The second half of this book gives an overview of some of the many choices in movement and sport available today. It is our attempt to provide a *representative* selection of physical training systems. It is only the tip of the iceberg and for every specific sport or discipline discussed there is another equally fulfilling.

The introduction to each section gives a bit of history to each category of movement. Each specific system, e.g. swimming or karate, is described briefly and then discussed in terms of which of the personal and physical goals, described in the first half of the book, it meets.

The purpose of this book is to provide you with the information, tools and self-knowledge to assist you in finding your individual route through the myriad movement forms, claims and the different choices offered in exercise today and so reach your own level of Stage Two fitness. Enjoy your journey!

PART ONE

Personal Goals

Health, Fitness and Well Being

Most of the research into the health benefits of exercise has concentrated on aerobic activity and its role in promoting cardiovascular fitness. This is largely because of the epidemic proportions of cardiovascular disease in the Western world. But scientists are starting to refocus their approach.

A debate between epidemiologists in *The Physician and Sports Medicine* in March 1985 emphasizes that physical activity is equally if not more important to health than cardiovascular fitness *per se*. Fitness tends to focus only on measurements of VO_2 Max (oxygen uptake). Physical activity takes into account energy expenditure, skeleto-muscular use, development of strength, flexibility and so on. All these elements play a part in maintaining health and preventing disease, including heart disease; fitness is not a simple matter of increasing oxygen uptake.

Running: the starting point

In 1971 Kenneth Cooper founded his Aerobics Centre in Dallas, Texas. Over 10,000 patients were evaluated, in the course of seven years, and followed medically supervised exercise programmes designed to deal with the problems of heart disease and obesity. His popularizing books, starting with *Aerobics* in 1968, began a massive grass roots movement in America towards jogging and running and other forms of aerobic activity.

While the last fifteen years have seen a 25 per cent drop in deaths from heart disease in the USA, death rates from cardiovascular disease (CHD) in Scotland and Ireland (with Finland) are now the highest in the world, with England and Wales following close behind. 1982 government statistics issued by the British Heart Foundation put the number of deaths under 75 years of age from heart disease at 140,500 a year. Heart disease attacks more men than women (although the gap is closing) and about 50 per cent of men in Britain today may develop major, minor, clinical or subclinical, chronic or passing CHD in middle age.

The major studies which influenced thinking on exercise in relation to heart disease, in addition to those of Kenneth Cooper, were those of epidemiologists (scientists who study the incidence of disease) Ralph Paffenbarger in San Francisco and J.N. Morris in London. Paffenbarger studied the health of 6351 dockworkers for over 25 years and found that those whose work was more physically demanding had roughly half the rate of heart disease. An even more impressive finding was that of the contrast in the rate of sudden deaths from heart disease: a ratio of one to three.

Professor Jerry Morris's now famous studies of bus conductors in the 1950s produced similar results. The conductors were less likely to suffer from heart disease than the drivers, simply because they walked up and down the stairs all day.

Paffenbarger followed his study of dockworkers with one on Harvard graduates in 1977. He compared their past records of physical activity and health when at university with their present levels of exercise, and noted their rate of death from heart disease. He found that those who took even a moderate amount of exercise each week were 64 per cent less at risk than their slothful contemporaries.

A recent study of leisure activity in civil servants by Morris showed that those civil servants who reported vigorous activity during their weekends also had a lower risk of heart attack. But one of the primary forms of activity undertaken was gardening – hardly thought of previously as vigorous enough to be of benefit to health.

Another significant conclusion was drawn by Ronald Laporte from Paffenbarger's Harvard alumni study. Paffenbarger's evidence that an additional 2000 calories should be expended to reduce the risk of heart disease was used as a basis of the recommendation to run 20 miles a week (since we use approximately 100 calories to run a mile). However, Laporte pointed out that this regime failed to take into account that this additional expenditure of 2000 calories a week *included* such daily activities as stair climbing, walking about the house or to work. In a recent study on post-menopausal women Laporte found that they expended 1200 calories a week mostly on walking and stair climbing; none of them ran.

Increased fitness usually accompanies increased activity but the growing consensus of opinion is that, first, milder levels of exercise are beneficial and, secondly, that all forms of exercise contribute to our overall health, and the health of our hearts.

Further research is beginning to suggest that it may well *not* be cardiovascular fitness that is the mediating link between activity and health. One of the major factors in decreasing heart disease risk is the reduction of levels of low-density lipoprotein cholesterol (LDL-C) and an increase in the level of high-density lipoprotein cholesterol (HDL-C), fat globules in the blood which have a scouring effect on the arteries. While aerobic exercise has been shown to raise the levels of HDL-C some studies show no significant change. Conversely weight training programmes (classed as anaerobic and so previously discounted as regards fitness) have been shown to raise HDL-C levels. This is an important concept in the relationship between exercise and health because if the crucial factor in cardiovascular health is not fitness (or increased VO_2Max) but raised HDL-C levels – which seem to be either hereditary or associated with high activity *generally* – then a reassessment of exercise patterns most beneficial to health must take place, and the over-emphasis on aerobic exercise might very well decrease.

There is already plenty of evidence to show that exercise is important for the health of the rest of the body, not just the cardiovascular system.

Exercise has been shown to be effective in countering the deterioration of muscle and bone which we tend to assume is an inevitable part of ageing. One English study showed that a programme of exercise prevented such deterioration over a period of ten years in a group of people aged between 54 and 71 years at the start of the study. Muscle deteriorates without use even in the young person. And further to this it loses some 30 per cent of its strength when its temperature drops by 5 degrees. A sedentary person, then, is in a weakened state, and doubly so when he gets cold. Add to this the loss of flexibility and decreased range of motion in the joints which goes with inactivity and one can see that this puts the older inactive person at especial risk. Bones also become more brittle with sedentary ageing. In fact bones begin to lose their calcium and other minerals even after a few days' bed-rest. Bone itself may soon start to be lost if the body is immobilised for very long periods. Known as osteoporosis, this process may be prevented by an active youth and also by regular exercise throughout one's life. One theory is that the anti-gravity musculature needs to be activated to prevent bone loss (so exercising lying down won't do!). At all events it is clear that exercise helps maintain health in people of all ages.

Weight control

One of the most vital aspects of exercise's contribution to health is its effectiveness in weight control.

Overweight and obesity are serious problems in the States and Britain. In 1983 the Royal College of Physicians published a report on obesity in which they stated that more than one third of all adults in Britain are overweight. And it appears we are getting fatter, this trend being particularly evident among young adults. The incidence of obesity is lower: six per cent of British men and eight per cent of women. Obesity is defined as the condition of being so overweight that the person runs immediate risks to his or her health.

In 1977 a committee of the US Senate chaired by George McGovern found in its report on dietary goals that nearly a quarter of the energy intake of the average American diet was in the form of sugar, and that fat made up a full 42 per cent of calorie intake. McGovern recommended cutting sugar by over half and fat by a third. The slack was to be taken up by an increase in starch (vegetables, rice, bread, potatoes) – a recommended increase from 22 to 48 per cent.

In Britain the evidence of the role of good food in keeping us out of the doctor's surgery, or worse, the surgeon's operating theatre, is only now being openly acknowledged and published for a lay public. This has come about following the NACNE report of 1983 which aimed at similar dietary reforms as the

McGovern Report and has met with similar obstruction from the food industry and other interested parties.

Weight control is achieved partly through a change in eating habits along NACNE lines: away from refined foods heavy in fats and sugars to whole foods, vegetables, fruit and cereals. But weight control is also a matter of energy balance. The Energy System (pages 58–71) explains the ways in which energy is stored and how and why fat is 'burned' by sustained exercise.

Professor Peter Wood, another pioneer in the health benefits of exercise, is the deputy director of the Stanford University Heart Disease Prevention Program, and initiator of a number of studies into the effects of running on health and obesity. While at first the experts refused to believe his results, what Wood proved has now become widely accepted: that regular runners could eat more and yet stay slimmer than their sedentary counterparts; that obesity is not so much a question of restricting calorie intake but of increasing through regular exercise the rate at which the body burns its fuel (the metabolic rate).

In one of Peter Wood's Stanford studies 48 sedentary middle-aged men took part in a one-year progressive exercise programme of walking, jogging and running. A control group agreed to remain sedentary. By the end of the year Wood found that the more miles the men ran each week, the more weight they lost; the more miles they ran, the more calories they reported eating, and the more they ate during the year, the greater the decrease in their body fat.

It appears that it is aerobic activity that is of particular benefit in weight control but any movement form performed regularly that offers the opportunity for vigorous activity over a period of about twenty minutes will have a beneficial effect. Another Stanford study found that middle-aged female tennis players, for example, were considerably slimmer (as well as fitter) and ate considerably more than the control group: an average of 2417 calories per day as opposed to 1490 calories.

The key to effective weight control, as with fitness, is regularity. A stop-start approach will not produce the training effects.

Lowered blood pressure is another benefit of regular aerobic exercise. Its opposite, high blood pressure or hypertension, is linked to another of the great health hazards talked about at great length today: stress. Other contributory factors to hypertension include a high-fat, high-sugar diet, genetic inheritance and lack of exercise.

Vigorous exercise can be highly effective in providing an outlet for the bottled up energy of a stressful day, where the anxiety of decision making, anger at the boss, or frustration with crowds on the underground, have found no release. At Cooper's institute he recommends that his staff and clients take their exercise at the end of the day for precisely this reason: he finds that letting off steam in a run or hard work-out is followed by relaxation and calm not only in measurements of the body systems, such as blood pressure and adrenalin levels, but also in their psychological outlook.

Well being

The documentation on the improvement to the body gained through exercise is now becoming mountainous. But there is a new criterion emerging in the exercise world in this Stage Two of the fitness scene: well being. Everyone talks about it but this improvement in emotional and psychological outlook is hard to measure. Well being is ultimately something personal and composed of many factors special to the individual. Slowly, physiological evidence is emerging that backs up the role of exercise in improving mental as well as physical health.

A study conducted by an American psychologist measured the benefits of running on his depressed patients both through standard personality tests and by using a control group. One group of patients was taken out running together for half an hour while members of the second group were individually given conventional analysis for an hour each. The tests showed a greater and faster improvement by the first group in their general sense of well being and in their control of anxiety and depression.

While Paffenbarger's dockworkers were no doubt protecting their hearts through their strenuous work, it is unlikely that they were expanding their overall sense of mental and physical health – their personal sense of well being – through this daily effort. Equally important is the need for a strong element of *play* in physical activity for it to be of real benefit to overall health.

For well being to be substantially increased, exercise must conform to three important principles: it must be recreational, not a chore; it must have an element of randomness, not just repetitive movement in it; and it must be chosen, not dictated.

Dyveke Spino began her career as a clinical psychologist, but was so impressed at the effects of exercise and movement over conventional psychoanalytic methods on depression and anxiety that she concentrated her work in that area, achieving particular success with women. She found that they gained in confidence and positive outlook as they began to move.

Apart from the increased self-respect which comes from employing one's will-power, the routine of physical exercise serves to create a stable, regular framework for what may be a fragmented lifestyle. Most of us experience from time to time that feeling of meaninglessness in our lives, or a sense of alienation from our environment. A demanding sports training schedule involving set timetables and goals for improvement each week can have a reassuring and validating effect.

Positive addiction

One of the main physiological reasons for the psychological benefits of exercise is that vigorous activity raises the endorphin levels in the body. Endorphins are the body's natural opiates, very similar in composition and effect to morphine. They can mask pain and help the body through times of strenuous activity. Thus the endorphin levels of pregnant women, for example, are naturally high, and even higher during delivery. There are many stories of a wounded soldier or injured marathoner who has not become aware of the pain until after the effort is passed. Cooper documents an Italian study conducted in 1980 which showed that endorphin levels in eight world-class athletes working to exhaustion on a treadmill rose over 500% above their level at rest when tested immediately after their effort. They were still above resting level half an hour afterwards.

Experiments have also shown that those who were out of condition had a more sustained rise in endorphin levels after completing a 12-minute exercise than those taking part who were already fit.

Endorphins are also the body's natural pain-killers. It is now emerging that just as the body becomes trained to higher levels of endurance or strength through vigorous activity so also it is trained to become used to, or even addicted, to higher endorphin levels. Researches are suggesting that this healthy addiction can gradually come to replace other, harmful addictions, such as smoking, excessive alcohol consumption, bingeing on sweets and chocolate, and over-eating generally.

There are dangers in this addiction to exercise. In 1983 a group of scientists from Arizona identified those most at risk as the middle-aged, highly competitive, goal-orientated man, saying that this group were so addicted to their run that they would exercise themselves to the point of collapse, and were in danger of permanently damaging muscles, tendons and bones. Tony Wilkinson in *The Listener* dubbed this fanaticism of the born-again runner 'Marathon Mentality'.

As always, physical and psychological go together and as a person experiences greater physical strength, improved flexibility or suppleness, more poise or balance, better circulation or coordination, so his perception of himself and his ability to act within his world will improve.

Health and well being have always been primary personal goals for anyone engaged in physical exercise. The pursuit of this goal requires you to consider seriously what *your* definition of health is and then make intelligent decisions based upon self-knowledge and a clear understanding of the physical goals you have established as your own. Don't take anyone else's definition of health – it is always a personal and relative state. Develop your acumen by educating yourself in your body's experience of well being and consciously choosing how you cultivate it. This is part of the whole process of Stage Two Fitness.

Creativity and Self-Expression

Nothing could be more immediately expressive of ourselves than our body movements. The language of the body, like any spoken language, can be learnt, refined, and used to communicate our feelings. Creativity involves the ability to show our individuality, so by becoming aware of our bodies we can learn to use them more expressively. This can be an immensely satisfying creative outlet. After the suppleness of babyhood and the free exploration of childhood, most of us start restricting our bodily movements to a small vocabulary and so our range of expression in that medium becomes very limited. In the same way we fail to develop the ability to interpret and appreciate the body language of others.

The rediscovery of our lost potential to express ourselves through movement is an exhilarating experience. It is often a major motivating factor in the individuals who seek out dance forms of movement. Dance is the most obviously creative of the movement forms whereas we tend to think of sport in terms other than expressive, artistic or creative.

One of the reasons these aspects of sport and exercise are often ignored is that in our culture creativity is conceived of as leading to a finished object: a painting, a play, a performance, a piece of music. It is harder for us to validate someone living or moving creatively when no obviously aesthetic production comes from their actions. We tend to see creativity as a process leading to an end which can be seen, heard or re-enacted again and again, rather than as an ongoing flow. We judge dance by what it looks like without taking into account that the creative experience as far as the dancer is concerned is primarily based on what it *feels* like.

It is not necessary to be a dancer to experience the creative aspect of physical movement. There are those who run or play tennis or swim for their health or because they think they ought to, and there are those for whom the activity is a direct expression of themselves, their way of being creative. For many martial artists, cross-country skiers, divers, as well as dancers, it is the attitude with which they perform their sport that counts. It is the level of awareness and focused concentration that gives activity its creative quality – and which also captivates the spectator.

Essentially any movement or exercise, from a yoga asana to a high-speed ski turn is beautiful to look at when performed with full attention, the refinement of skill and the ease of practised execution. It was the apparent effortlessness of Torvill and Dean's 'Bolero' which captured the imagination of the onlooker.

There is much talk now of the 'kinaesthetic experience'. This important concept emphasized by leading thinkers in movement and sports today is helping to shift the focus from results, or production – what you have to show for your endeavour – to the experience of doing. While the aesthetic refers to what something looks like, how, for instance, movement is experienced by the spectator, the kinaesthetic refers to how we feel doing the movement, the quality and beauty of the experience for the mover.

This is a valuable shift in emphasis. It suggests that all of us can potentially experience ourselves as creative individuals, not just the rare few, the artists, dancers, performers, and star athletes among us. Emphasis on the kinaesthetic also further encourages the shift in awareness to what is taking place inside us, how we *feel* doing things, rather than judging the means by the results. Sensitivity to inner energy is central to the martial arts; it is no accident that they are referred to as 'arts' rather than sports.

Those who have been involved in sport and movement all their lives, or those who teach, frequently express the creative aspect. Percy Wells Cerutty, the great Australian running coach, said: 'Running as I teach it is not a sport of physical activity so much as a concentration of expression of ourselves, physical, mental, and spiritual.'

Preparing the body for movement is an important part of movement as a creative process. The person who rushes into a game of football, or leaps straight into a fast run, or jumps into an aerobics class right off the street, risks not only injury but is also denied the mental and emotional induction into the aesthetic pleasure of activity. It's like going to the opera but missing the overture which introduces the themes to be fully expressed in the body of the work.

All professional athletes and dancers undertake careful warm-up sessions – they prepare themselves. This is to warm the muscles and tone the body before exertion in order to lessen the risk of injury, but since body and mind are one continuum, by slowly warming and opening ourselves physically we are also expanding and 'tuning' our other senses. We are sensitizing our body, tuning up as any artist does.

One of the most elegant accounts of creativity is the book *The Courage to Create* by psychologist Rollo May. In one passage May talks about the need for receptivity in the creative act and the ability required of the artist to be open and to wait:

> An artist's waiting is not to be confused with laziness or passivity. It requires a great degree of attention, as when a diver is poised on the end of the springboard, not jumping but holding his or her muscles in sensitive balance for the right second. It is an active listening, keyed to hear the answer, alert to see whatever can be glimpsed when the vision or the words do come . . . it is necessary that the artist has this sense of tuning, that he or she respect these periods of receptivity as part of the mystery of creativity and creation. (page 81)

For 'artist' we can substitute athlete. Team players and solo stars alike will recognize the quality of these moments, when everything is hyper-tuned for action, like a lion, every muscle coiled ready to spring, waiting only for the exact second. These are the qualities often identified as 'peak experiences' by sports people. Billie Jean King writes in her autobiography: 'It's a perfect combination of . . . violent action taking place in an atmosphere of total tranquillity . . . When it happens I want to stop the match and grab the microphone and shout, "*That's what it's all about*" . . .'

For centuries the mind has received a great deal of attention, the body treated as a mere vehicle or adjunct. The interconnection between the two has been generally ignored. Sport and movement forms can provide a medium for the interplay between mind and body, and help to bring the two into greater harmony. This is what we witness in the athletes and dancers we admire – Nureyev, Bjorn Borg, Daley Thompson, Torvill and Dean. When mind and body are totally focused, working together as a whole, the full reserves of creative energy (which we all of us have within us), are released and self-expression becomes the creative act. The kinaesthetic and the aesthetic experiences merge to become one and the same.

In his book, *Beyond Jogging*, Mike Spino takes this a step further:

> I see running as an art form, as well as a means of physical conditioning. A blending of the power of the body and mind can carry us to new plateaus of creative achievement . . . Jogging is not enough. In a society that seeks new paradigms

in many aspects of living, the goal for the athlete is to offer a new model of creativity and insight through sport.

Creativity is the resolution of hitherto unrelated or conflicting parts into an harmonious whole. Nowhere is that more clearly manifested than in the relationship between body, mind, emotions and spirit. Sport, dance, martial arts, *all* offer the possibility for this creative synthesis to take place.

Social Factors

Sport is one of the great integrating elements in our society. It crosses cultural and racial boundaries and draws together men and women from different backgrounds, ages, races, creeds, political views and beliefs. More television time and newspaper pages are devoted to sports coverage than to any other single subject, and billions of pounds, dollars, Deutschmarks and yen are spent promoting sport, building facilities and organizing events for spectators.

One of the main reasons behind the power of sport over our imaginations, and the draw to so many of us to participate in some form of organized physical activity, is that the world of sport is a world apart from that of everyday life. Johan Huizinga, the Dutch historian and author of the 1938 classic and definitive study, *Homo Ludens*, defines play as: '. . . a voluntary activity or occupation executed within fixed limits of time and place according to rules freely accepted but absolutely binding, having its aim in itself and accompanied by a feeling of tension, joy and the consciousness that it is "different" from "ordinary life".' Understanding and accepting the rules of a given game gives one a sense of belonging. There is nothing so lonely as being the odd one out in a crowd of cricket lovers swapping statistics, or a bunch of rugby players recounting epic tales. And there is nothing so warming as being a part of a group engaged in the same sport or game. The importance of having that separate world, apart from the business of daily life, where a different and simpler set of rules pertain (rules that we all adhere to in the common aim of playing the game), cannot be over-emphasized.

As a socializing force, play is pre-eminent throughout history.

Children in primitive hunting and gathering tribes would imitate their elders in the hunt, and even in contemporary Eskimo tribes in Greenland children make small bows and arrows and spears in their play hunting games. Later, in the real hunt, the socializing force of these childhood games is proven when the young adolescent is able to merge with the subtle rhythms of the hunting party. In many primitive cultures, transition from childhood through puberty to adulthood is marked by ritual games and dances and in every society ritualized hunts and games were acted out in drama and dance. In *The Iliad*, to commemorate the death of Patroclus, the Greeks stopped combat and put on funeral games as a rite of passage. The original Olympian games were far more than opportunities for individuals to express their prowess in their chosen sport; they were a ritual celebration dedicated to the gods and to the ideal of 'manhood'.

Long before Dr Thomas Arnold, headmaster of Rugby Public School (which gave its name to the game) appeared on the scene, sport had been a major force for social integration among these British schoolchildren. The boys organized their own games of football, hunting and cricket in a passionate if lawless way. Arnold himself hated football and was only mildly interested in cricket, gymnastics and spear-throwing! What he was responsible for was putting some law and order into the games and integrating them into the school's curriculum.

So what began as an instinctive and self-regulating system of games based on the essence of play, became, according to a contemporary government report of 1864, not merely exercise but a method of building 'character', 'moral fibre' and 'some of the most valuable social qualities and manly virtues'. In the same way as the traditions of prefects and punishments were incorporated into the fabric of public school life, and from there into the whole British educational system, so sports were also a way of incorporating newcomers into the social structure. At their best, organized school games provided an opportunity for camaraderie, inclusion and the inspiration of team spirit. At their worst they became a brutal and mindless means by which authority and social norms were imposed unfeelingly and unilaterally with the ulterior moral justification of being 'for your own good'.

In Sweden, where sport is not forced on children as part of the official education process, the social as well as the health benefits of recreational exercise are better recognized and valued, and recreational sports become a life-long part of daily living. The social side is strong. One in six Swedes belongs to at least one community sports centre and 60 per cent of all Swedish children between the ages of seven and eighteen belong to sports clubs. According to a study reported in *The Physician and Sports Medicine*, competitive sports are organized so as not to be restrictive or exclusive; having a good time and the development of skills are the goals. A great deal of government money is directed into sports research – 52 projects were funded in 1981, which for a country of only 8 million people is impressive. But more importantly, because the research findings are widely disseminated and are shared with the general public, not just with elite athletes, sports science is demythologized, and the health benefits reinforce the social inclinations of a sporty people.

The great misfortune of arbitrarily imposed sport is that far from proving to be a uniformly successful socializing force, it often provokes a backlash, particularly in schoolchildren, against authority and against sport in general. In addition, self-esteem takes a severe blow (sometimes never overcome) from the experience of failure to achieve within the restricted options of the sports curriculum. The result may make the individual steer clear of sports from then on, missing out on the more personal joys and the pleasure of sporting camaraderie. For it is on the level of personal relationships and the interaction between fellow participants on a team that the social plusses of physical training break through. And this is characteristic of all physical training environs, from the exercise studio to the martial arts dojo, from the yoga class to the football pitch.

A woman runner who began to run regularly with the Serpentine Runners Club in Hyde Park, at first strictly for her own well being, describes the shift that took place:

Growing up in the 1960s we were a bit sniffy about the camaraderie of sporty groups – what we used to call the 'hoorays' at university. All that hale-fellow-well-met stuff, hugging and back slapping, and the apparent aimlessness of the conversation, made up largely of in-jokes, in-anecdotes and in-teasing. But over the years of my membership with the

SRC the original motivation was superseded by a more important and, for me, surprising recognition. It was no longer only the running in itself which kept me going to the SRC. It was the quality of companionship and warmth which I found there that drew me – and others – back again and again. It is a friendliness that has nothing to do with who you are or what you do or have achieved in the outside world, nothing to do with how clever or attractive you may be, nothing to do with social status or money. We are simply all runners, together because we like to run.

At its best the closeness and mutual acceptance that builds up in running groups, in teams and in clubs for all kinds of physical activities is similar in kind to the supportive love that we experience (if we are lucky) as children from our parents .

But in the same way as our parents' love depends on us being part of the family group and on the tacit acceptance of its rules, so the togetherness we feel in the sports group depends on us accepting the rules of the game. If you were to stop suddenly in the middle of a run and say 'this is silly, I'm going home', or if you were suddenly to take a short cut for no justifiable reason, you would soon find yourself receiving a chilly shoulder from the rest of the group. Indeed one founder member of the SRC, much loved by everyone for his jokey and kindly personality, and a leading light in the Club's activities, was found to have started on the Isle of Dogs to cut half an hour off his time in the 1983 London Marathon. The reaction of the Club was one of horror and disgust, and despite the years of sharing that had gone before, the frozen reception the Club now gave him forced him to resign forthwith.

The social element of sport is a big attraction for the vast majority who take up recreational exercise, and many clubs and sports centres now emphasize this aspect with bars and cafés, discos and other events which draw in the rest of the family to the activity group.

Togetherness and love is something we are rather shy about in Britain. We tend not to express our appreciation or love of others easily and openly, and we touch less than any other nation. All this changes in the context of sports and exercise. Previously reserved people start hugging each other, a fellow exerciser is quick to place a friendly corrective hand on back or shoulder, and a muscle massage becomes the norm after some runs or classes. And the celebration and fellow feeling after a goal on the football field is well known. It was said by one American sports commentator that 'nothing except war brings men closer together than professional sports.'

The sense of togetherness is particularly strong in team sports. Team spirit grows as a group of men or women play together, a spirit which can be more binding and powerful than any other aspect of the game. One American football player expressed this feeling: 'We're all different . . . and yet we all go down the same road, hand in hand . . . no individual on this club will go directly against another's feelings, no matter what his own opinion is . . . I guess it all comes down to consideration . . . or love.' And another said: I've never seen any place in the world, any human activity, where love is more exemplified than on the pro football field. You go through so much together.'

A sense of comradeship, togetherness, love, warmth, shared fun. How many leisure occupations can offer these? For those of us, particularly, who live alone in big cities, who work in large organizations where the only sharing that goes on is passing an accounts slips from one in-tray to another, the social aspects of exercise can be a life-saver. Alienation and fragmentation are peculiarly common twentieth century diseases and most of us suffer from these feelings some of the time: joining the thronging hordes on the ride to work in the morning, grey faces, no one speaking to anyone else; or the mother living in a high rise with small children and anonymous neighbours; the harried boss with so many responsibilities and anxieties he feels pulled in all directions. The undemanding community feeling and easy warmth of a sports group can provide just the balancer needed.

Stephen Van Dyke, the youngest skipper in the 1969 Transatlantic race felt there were greater rewards than trophies: 'I'm not hellbent on winning. I want . . . a feeling of having met a singular challenge with my crew . . . . That was the greatest sense of comradeship I've ever experienced.'

Challenge and Power

Sport has long been recognized as one field where our need to meet challenges and express our personal power can be given free expression. The philosopher Nietzche maintained that the will to power can only be expressed against obstacles and so we therefore deliberately search out things that resist us. Mountain climbing, surfing, motor racing and other sports in which the individual pits him or herself against the forces of nature are supreme examples of this urge. The challenge is intrinsic in all physical exercise to a lesser or greater degree: the challenge of testing one's strength and endurance in a long run, the challenge of running faster than a companion or faster than one's own previous time, the challenge of a match, a jump, a game in which we find ourselves pitted against some obstacle, tangible or intangible. The element is always there if we choose to recognize it and it is through meeting such challenges that we experience our personal power.

The interaction with others and the environment play an integral part in the discovery of personal power, which extends to a sense of controlling more than just oneself. The mountaineer Chris Bonnington describes this process:

> With experience one gains greater control. This led to a real pleasure in a struggle with the elements at their worst – certainly my most memorable, and in a way most enjoyable, days climbing have been in violent storms in the Alps, when the wind and snow have torn at my anorak-covered body; when my wits and judgement have been extended to the full and yet, in spite of all, I have remained on top of the situation.

We experience this power, sometimes almost by surprise, as a result of our efforts. Bruce Jenner, speaking of his performance in the decathlon at the 1976 Olympics:

> . . . a strange feeling began to come over me. In four events so far, I'd set three personal bests and come within a couple hundredths of my electronic p.r. (personal record) in the hundred. I started to feel that there was nothing I couldn't do if I had to. It was a feeling of awesome power, except that I was in awe of myself, knocking off these p.rs. just like that. I was rising above myself, doing things I had no right to be doing.

Being best is a deeply ingrained concept in Anglo-Saxon culture. Ted Williams, one of America's greatest baseball players, said of the game: 'Baseball gives every American boy a chance to excel, not just to be as good as someone else but to be better than someone else. This is the nature of man and the nature of the game.' And British racing driver Graham Hill was even more categorical about his sport: 'That's the whole point of racing, really, to prove you're the best. If you don't believe it, then you're prepared for defeat, aren't you.'

Competitiveness and personal power are so inextricably intertwined that we sometimes become myopically fixed on the goal of winning. Grantland Rice, a famous American sports broadcaster of several decades ago, is still renowned for his oft-quoted pronouncement; 'It's not whether you win or lose, but how you play the game.' Vince Lombardi, the legendary coach of American football team, the Green Bay Packers, had another perspective – 'Winning isn't everything; it's the only thing.' Or as Gene Autry, former Hollywood cowboy and owner of the California Angels Baseball Club, put it rather more bluntly: 'Well, Grantland Rice can go to hell, as far as I'm concerned.'

Competition is all pervasive in our society. Considering the economic remuneration which follows from successful competition not only in professional sport but in all areas of life, it is idealistic to say that one should simply play the game beautifully or at the worst restrict competition to the sanitised areas of sport. That's not the way it works out.

D.H. Lawrence felt strongly that sport was the right and proper field for competitiveness between men to be expressed, rather than in the area of work where we should be interacting in harmony. He wanted the reinstatement of gymnasia as places of 'fierce, unrelenting, honourable contest'. Roger Bannister, on the other hand, sees sport as primarily a testing ground for life itself, a place where a man proves himself to be 'a true man'. This attitude has been echoed by many a headmaster, teacher, coach and old boy: 'The battle of Waterloo was won on the playing fields of Eton'.

But while it is fine to propose, like Lawrence, that aggression, competition and the contest of personal power should be segregated and restricted to the playing fields, Wellington's now hackneyed comment bears a closer resemblance to the way things are. The advantage of the sporting situation is that it does provide a socially acceptable arena where the sometimes submerged and distorted impulses to aggression and conflict can be expressed within tightly constructed guidelines and parameters of safety. The possibility open to individuals in such situations is that through meeting the challenge of a competition or of a mountain climb, they will experience not only the positive expression of their aggressive drive and all of its emotional concommitants but they will also begin to contact their own sense of personal power. Through meeting the challenge they in turn meet themselves and what they are capable of bringing to that challenge.

All of us from time to time and in different situations need the challenge of the competitor or the obstacle in order to draw the best out of ourselves. So it is a fine line we must tread, between an addiction to neurotic competitiveness and the other extreme of playing only in order to play 'beautifully', thus annulling the parameters, or rules, of the game.

Timothy Gallwey, amateur tennis player and author of *The Inner Game*, explored this dilemma. He tells the story of losing the All-American Junior Championships when he was fifteen, because, at two sets to love up, he suddenly felt sorry for the eighteen year old he was about to beat: 'If I assume that I am making myself more worthy of respect by winning, then I must believe, consciously or unconsciously, that by defeating someone, I am making him less worthy of respect.'

Neurotic competitiveness then, is when the player is not interested in playing the game, only in the attention and respect he will gain from winning. But, as John Syer concludes in *Sporting Body, Sporting Mind*, competitiveness is not necessarily neurotic:

A true competitor, a competitor who is creative and who is interested in the game, is not competing to prove he is something he feels he should be, *but to find out who he really is*, in the faith that whoever or whatever that turns out to be; it will be unique and perfect. (Our italics.)

Gallwey himself came to realize this truth in relation to the surfer waiting for the big wave:

It is only against the *big* waves that the surfer is required to use all his skill, all his courage and concentration to overcome; only *then* can he realize the true limits of his capacities. (Our italics.)

In other words, the more challenging the obstacle that the surfer or the runner, or the tennis player, faces, the greater the opportunity for discovering and extending *true* potential.

Self-validation, as opposed to needing the approval of an outside authority, is one of the most central aspects of this personal power. This deep self-confidence comes by way of choosing a sport or exercise usually for some profound but often indefinable reason that has something to do with the sheer *joy* of doing it. If our goal is narrowly definable – such as to lose weight, to win the competition, to look better than our neighbours – then our outlook and experiences will be similarly narrow; and so will the rewards we gain from the activity.

On the whole, those who take up exercise from obligation, guilt, self-denial or simply to win, rarely stick at it. Joy is absent, the activity is another chore. And it is hard to feel proud and in touch with one's free spirit in such circumstances. The running coach Percy Wells Cerutty made this point forcefully in relation to his work with professional athletes:

> If the athlete is not a free and full worker, working him to a fixed schedule, or according to the dictate of another person, such as a coach or authority, must end in confusion, disappointment, disillusionment, partial successes to what they might have been, breakdown and eventual frustrations and abandonment.

Cerutty's grim warning applies to us all – professional or casual exerciser. Unless an activity is freely undertaken because you want to do it, for yourself, then eventually the effort will get to you, and the most likely result will be that either you will drop the activity or it will drop you. A great many sports injuries amongst casual exercisers are the result of a half-hearted involvement.

When we commit ourselves, and are fully with the experience of the sport, martial art or movement form chosen then we can begin to realize our potential. Power and self-fulfilment are concepts that transcend competition. In essence when we take up a challenge we are confronting ourselves: 'Can I do it?' This is the question each of us faces as we prepare for a run, a jump, the rock face, or the match.

Freedom and Self-Mastery

As we begin to experience personal power we move towards the sense of freedom and autonomy that accompany it. We can say: When I not only experience control of myself but also freedom from fruitless comparisons with others and measurements based on social expectations, I connect with an inner sense of independence which becomes identified with self-mastery and autonomy.

As a concept, self-mastery, belongs, in Western fantasy, to the world of Samurai warriors and Zen monks. Yet as an experience in sport, dance, body conditioning and martial arts it is not only real but tangible. In a society which exercises its influence over our psyches through advertising, marketing, legislation and the media – quite apart from the socialising controls which take place in childhood, in school and through peer groups – it is a tremendously liberating experience to achieve a degree of self-mastery. This is not the arbitrary exercise of will-power over oneself but the self-recognition which is experienced as the result of one's own efforts.

The feeling can occur in any sport or activity. One of the joys of physical training, be it for a downhill skiing competition, or at the local gym on an evening workout, is to experience the change we create in our body and in its performance. And when we create changes in our physical bodies, we create change in our mental and emotional states as well. Roger Bannister says of the sportsman that he is seeking 'the deep satisfaction, the sense of personal dignity which comes when the body and mind are fully coordinated and they have achieved mastery over themselves'.

Although the concept of self-mastery is traditionally a masculine one, participation in sports and simple exercise programmes has helped women to reshape their own image as well. As a woman discovers mastery over her physical body she need no longer conceive of herself as a passive object, to be compared, judged, admired or found wanting both by herself and others. Self image shifts from being an outside-in process of looking at mirror, advert or magazine model and seeing how one matches up, to being an inside-out process, of sensing one's strength, the pleasure and pain of direct experience and an ability to shape oneself and one's world.

For both men and women, in the face of a world increasingly, it seems, outside our control, the experience of self-mastery through controlled and regular physical training is more than invigorating. The measure of satisfaction and self-confidence gained can have significant repercussions in all areas of our lives.

Self-mastery is the result of consistency. It is not an elusive concept; and it is not bestowed from on high by god or guru. It involves how we choose to be and how we present ourselves to the world. By taking action – literally by just moving in a physical and purposeful way – we are not only expressing ourselves but changing ourselves. We become stronger, fitter or more supple; we become more graceful, centred or effortless; we may practise yoga or we may weight train. It is precisely through choosing and deciding that we shape our bodies and lives. Every day is made up of a mass of little decisions, as simple as whether or not to eat an apple or have coffee or tea, or as critical as whether to buy more shares of a company, to spend money on a new car, or save it up. If the factors which determine these and other critical decisions are outside of my control then I experience myself as being 'at effect' instead of 'at cause'. I react to things rather than initiate.

In her research on Biofeedback, Dr Barbara Brown stresses the crucial importance of where the individual experiences his or her 'locus of control'. In other words, do you experience the factors which shape your life, the ways you express yourself, and the choices open to you, as being inside yourself, and under your control, or outside yourself, vested in the world, the environment, the control of other people? The question remains, however: how do I achieve this inner self-control?

The crux of the matter is clarified in Italian psychiatrist Roberto Assagioli's description of the 'will' as distinct from 'will-power'. Will-power, he says, is what you use to push a car up a hill; using the will, however, might entail *choosing* to push, driving the car, asking for assistance or otherwise directing the car up the hill. Many of us experience our lives as one long process of pushing cars up hills – everything is a struggle, things weigh us down, and for all our strenuous efforts we seem to get nowhere. When we use our will consciously, on the other hand, we have a sense of seeing the situation or problem clearly, of being able to assess what is needed and which course of action to take. We are in control, and we can choose whether to act or not.

One of the most attractive aspects of exercise and sport is the discipline involved. Unfortunately the word conjures images of the British stiff upper lip, rigid backbone and short sharp shocks. But the kind of discipline we are talking about here is the self-imposed kind, owing more to Zen than the Union Jack, more to skill than brute strength. The discipline experienced in self-mastery gives you a sense of freedom and autonomy, not the rigid control which is inhibiting and limited.

To make this more clear, Assagioli distinguishes between the 'strong will' – the blood-and-guts all-out effort – and the 'skilful will' – using the amount of energy necessary to accomplish the task without over-exertion. It takes a great deal of strong will *and* skilful will to complete a marathon or a triathlon. The right combination of effort sustained throughout the race with the appropriate pacing and the appropriate burst of speed or extra effort at crucial moments combine to produce the result.

But Assagioli makes an even more important point. Through the judicious use of our will we begin to contact that part of ourselves which actually does the choosing. Call it the 'I', that part of me which can choose to train myself physically on a regular and testing programme, that can *choose* to regularize my diet, that can *choose* to take a new job which is more satisfying, and the part of me which can *choose* to lie in on a lazy Sunday morning because I want and need the rest. We begin to make not only immediate decisions more clearly, but begin to participate consciously in mapping out the longer-term course of our lives.

Choice becomes something that is nourishing, bound up with pleasure and with doing good to oneself, and for oneself. Self-mastery is a part of the maturing process, of learning that control and organization are necessary foundations for all true freedom. But even more: making conscious choices enables us to align our actions with our unfolding purpose. The ability to really choose gives us the opportunity to become who we right and truly are.

Achievement and the Search for Perfection

As we watch the superb athlete, in admiration of his feats, we sometimes catch a glimpse of that towards which he aspires: perfection. In *Sport and Identity*, Peter Neal pursues this idea: 'Sport has remained an attraction to thousands and millions because it exemplifies man's search for perfection . . . it allows glimpses of what man is, but also of what he could be.'

The desire for achievement and the search for perfection are closely linked to the challenge of self-mastery and the thirst for power. But while power involves the testing of one's strength against others or an obstacle, and self-mastery is concerned with self-regulation or control, the desire to achieve and a striving for perfection imply measuring oneself against a standard beyond yourself and others. And as the ancient Greeks knew, in facing ourselves in this way, we face our very mortality – and defy it. The sporting prowess of the ancient Greek heroes – exemplified in the Olympics – was both in imitation of the gods and a challenge to them. In extending ourselves beyond our limits we become, of only for a moment, immortal.

There is a distinction to be made between wanting to achieve and seeking perfection. Research from the Institute for the Study of Athletic Motivation in the USA showed that of a sample of 15,000 athletes, those who survived the high drop-out rate in competitive sport displayed a number of salient characteristics. The need for achievement came top of the list. But second only to this was that they 'set high but realistic goals for themselves'. Realistic is the key word. High achievement motivation is essential for optimal sports performance. But perfection, as the Jungian analyst, Marian Woodman, points out in her brilliant study *Addiction to Perfection*, is the preserve of the gods. It is a super-human quality, so to strive after perfection will always carry within it the seeds of defeat. We will always necessarily fall short of an unattainable goal.

Taking part in sport and physical activities can give us the experience of achievement often quite out of proportion to the objective value of the accomplishment. Runners, for example, frequently tell their story of fighting through exhaustion, the troubles of the day or their body's reluctance in their evening run . . . to get to the end of that five miles, heart pounding, sweat pouring and feeling the glow of pride, the satisfaction of achievement. Yet in real terms it is a small thing. Gill Hudson, ex-editor of *Fitness* magazine, runs in the morning. 'After my couple of miles I feel so pleased with myself. I feel that however the rest of the day goes, I've already achieved something.' All for two miles!

We all hold our own notion of what constitutes perfection as a goal we strive for, consciously or unconsciously. Young skaters today, for instance, strive to be the next Torvill and Dean. It does not matter that they will never achieve that aim, just as no two people are ever alike. They may achieve acclaim of their own, but they will never repeat the identical accomplishments. Likewise, even though we may consider the skating stars' performance to be perfection incarnate, they themselves are doubtless not only aware of a hundred little faults, but are also aiming at their own image of perfection – always just beyond.

In his book, *Meaning in Movement, Sport and Physical Education*, Peter Arnold makes a useful grouping of physical activities into the following three categories:

1. Sports activities, such as tennis, golf, athletics, in which the goal is specifically independent of the means of achieving it.
2. Activities in which the ends and means go together: gymnastics, diving, skating and skiing. In competition the athlete is judged on the actual performance rather than achieving a final goal, or winning against another player as in the first category.
3. Activities in which it is illogical to talk of a distinction of ends and means in the first place: dance, some martial arts, exercise classes, yoga. In these exercise forms no goal is being aimed for, the achievement is in the individual's sense of doing the exercise well.

All these categories contain the element of achievement and an image of perfection to be sought, and in all we can experience those magical moments, when we feel 'Yes, that was it – perfect!'. But they are quite different in kind and will elicit quite different qualities and types of effort from the individual.

Those people with a strong goal orientation, to whom it matters to win and to beat an opponent, will be more attracted to the first two categories, and those for whom achievement and perfection reside in the focus and concentration of the slower and non-competitive activities, will be drawn to the last category, to those movement forms which carry a high artistic and kinaesthetic content.

One of the pitfalls of searching after perfection lies in the avoidance of outright competition. It is a myth, supported by an overly sentimental Western view of Eastern philosophy that one has only to seek perfection and stay above the fray of the common masses. Timothy Gallwey, after a loss in the finals of the US Junior Tennis Championship said:

> I became non-competitive. Instead of trying to win, I decided to attempt only to play beautifully and excellently . . . absorbed solely in achieving excellence for its own sake. But something was missing, I didn't experience a desire to win and, as a result, I often lacked the necessary determination.

It's one thing to *talk* about perfection but if our opponent chases us all over the tennis court or leaves us in a cloud of dust it is rather hard to speak in all honesty of 'achievement'.

Perfection is an ideal, the possession of the gods, and yet it is in the attempt to translate our conceptions of perfection into reality that we actually experience glimpses of what it is all about. Yuri Vlasov, the champion Russian weightlifter describes such an experience:

> At the peak of tremendous and victorious effort . . . while the blood is pounding in your head, all suddenly becomes quiet within you. Everything seems clearer and whiter than ever before, as if great spotlights had been turned on. At that moment you have the conviction that you contain all the power in the world, that you are capable of everything, that you have wings. There are no more precious moments in life than this, the white moment, and you will work very hard for years just to taste it again.

Kathrine Switzer, the first woman marathoner, completing the Boston marathon in 1967, brings this ecstasy back to earth: 'You look back over the miles and miles you've run and think, I did that! – You never feel the same about yourself again.'

Unity

Our era is now witnessing the beginnings of what will become a profound and hopefully enduring shift away from a culture of dominance to one of dominion, away from separation to union. The fact that the heritage of our spiritual and material fragmentation is actually quite recent doesn't make it any less confusing or the distortions any less painful and ugly. Some people signal Descartes, and his 'I think, therefore I am', as the beginning of the separation into mind and body. Others pin it on Aristotle's working axiom: either something is A, or it is not A. Medieval Christianity used this as a basis to contend that body and spirit are separate entities. But whatever the cause, as our world has become more and more fragmented and torn so the hunger for unity has grown into starvation: we are ravenous for a connection with some greater whole. Oscar Wilde puts this disparity beautifully in his essay *De Profundis*:

> It seems to me that we all look at Nature too much, and live with her too little. I discern great sanity in the Greek attitude. They never chattered about sunsets, or discussed whether the shadows on the grass were mauve or not. But they saw that the sea was for the swimmer and the sand was for the feet of the runner. They loved the trees for the shadow they cast, and the forest for the silence at noon.

Now, politically, socially and personally, individuals are beginning to realize that through cooperation and unity with nature not only is our experience of ourselves enhanced but that our very survival may depend upon this increased empathy, understanding and tolerance. Morehei Uyeshiba, the founder of aikido taught:

> The secret of aikido is to harmonize ourselves with the movement of the universe and bring ourselves into accord with the universe itself. He who has gained the secret of aikido has the universe in himself and can say: 'I am the universe.' I am never defeated, however fast the enemy may attack . . . When the enemy tries to fight with him, the universe itself, he has to break the harmony of the universe. Hence at the moment he has the mind to fight with me, he is already defeated.

We are coming to terms with the fact that being dominant over your own bodies is a dead end. You can only push and force your body so far and then it rebels. There is now a growing shift towards a co-creative relationship with our bodies.

This new outlook is taking place on several levels within the exercise field. The vogue for hard-edged aerobics classes is giving way to gentler, all-round body conditioning routines. And at the popular level of the fitness routines of the stars, Jane Fonda's workout book was followed in late 1984 by Raquel Welch's formula. Her book, written with the same compelling conviction and sincerity as Fonda's decries the tough cookie image of the workout boom. Welch put her name behind the non-violent but highly disciplined approach of yoga – at a time when yoga was far from being in the limelight. As Welch disarmingly puts it, if you treat your own body in an unforgiving way then that is probably how you will treat the world around you. Yoga is based on the concept of unity, the 'yoking' together of sun and moon, or in Western terms, of the active, masculine drive with passive, feminine receptivity.

The same shift away from dominance is happening in the religious and spiritual sphere. We in the West are inheritors of the Judeo-Christian ethic of spirit as transcendent and with it the attitude that the flesh is earthly, base and must therefore be subjected for the spirit to free itself and achieve grace and unity with God. From this comes the tradition of punishing the body, dominating it, of putting it through stringent workout and purification routines. Another approach to worship, recognized by some Eastern religions such as Taoism, and our pagan forebears, sees the spirit and religious energy as within the earth, within Nature and within the body. The gradual but steady rise in the West of participation in yoga and the martial arts as well as interest in Eastern religions reflects the search for more unifying concepts.

The concept of blending or unifying with the natural forces around you is central to the martial arts. It extends even to merging with your opponent as one judo manual explains: 'You and your opponent will no longer be two bodies separated physically from each other but a single entity, physically, mentally, and spiritually inseparable. Therefore, the motion of your opponent may be considered your motion. And you can lure him to any posture you like and effectively apply a large force on him. You can throw him as easily as you can yourself.'

The experience of unity is not only found in the practice of martial arts or yoga. Surfers and skiers talk of the oneness they experience with the curling wave or the white slope. Runners, often as they near the point of exhaustion, experience an alteration in their perceptions and suddenly feel a surge of new energy that may enter them from the cheers of the crowd urging them on in a race, or a sense of blending into the forces of the landscape around them in a solo run. And some athletes feel a sense of unity with their equipment, a racing driver with his car, a pilot with his plane.

In his book, *The Psychic Side of Sports*, Michael Murphy cites numerous examples of altered states of perception and experiences of unity amongst athletes. A sometime philosopher, Murphy co-founded the famous Esalen Institute in California which has remained at the leading edge of the field of humanistic psychology and experimentation in psychic phenomena. Murphy, with others like running coach Mike Spino and author George Leonard, has explored human potential in particular through sports. Their books have done much to disseminate and popularize the confirmed beliefs of professional athletes – hitherto kept relatively secret – that sport is about a lot more than just physical strength and skill or pushing the body to achieve a goal. These experiences can be frightening if only because they are so foreign and bear so little relationship to our everyday sense of what constitutes reality, of the laws of the possible.

Murphy recounts the story of Bob Beamon when he broke the long jump record at the Mexico Olympics by two feet (a record unequalled since). It was only some minutes later, after he had put on his track suit, that Beamon realized the enormity of what he had done: he fell to his knees, clasping his head in his hands, nausea overcoming him. 'Tell me I am not dreaming', was all he could mumble, and later said that if he had had high blood pressure he would have had a stroke.

In meditation, the silent reciting of a single word, or mantra, has the effect of quieting the mind to allow our awareness of things other than our own thoughts to expand. There are certain exercise forms that will expressly encourage a meditative state more than others. These are the martial arts, in particular the slower, less attacking forms such as t'ai-chi and aikido. Some forms of movement awareness and rhythmic dance may also induce a receptive and relaxed state. In sports, running with its repetitive movement creates for some an almost trance-like state of heightened awareness. Running can also bring you into a close contact with nature and an intimacy with the changing weather and seasons, a sense of harmony and oneness with the universe.

Dr George Sheehan, author of several popular books on running, describes the different stages of a run. The first 30 minutes are for his body, the joy of physical ability, feeling in control, thinking out the problems of the day:

> What lies beyond this fitness of muscle? I can only answer for myself. The next 30 minutes is for my soul. In it, I come upon the third wind (unlike the second wind, which is physiological). And then I see myself not as an individual, but as part of the universe. In it, I can happen upon anything I ever read or saw or experienced. Every fact and instinct and emotion is unlocked and made available to me through some mysterious operation in my brain.

We are into an area which is subjective, for the most part unverifiable, and so, for some, 'weird' and offputting. Sports as a transcendant experience is not for everyone. The pragmatist can choose a quite different approach and if he so chooses he can be sure that no bizarre happenings will disturb his training routine. The truth is – at least in the West – that our exploration into the psychic side of sports is still very young and tentative. We hardly even have the language to speak about such experiences, and most healthy, strong athletes, or ordinary people who just want to exercise to get fit shy away from this 'third man'. Or else they are embarrassed to talk about their deeply subjective feelings, to talk of a sense of unity and oneness with the natural world, the sense of floating above it all, of suddenly acquiring powers they never thought they had.

And yet at some level this is what we are all seeking – those magic moments when suddenly everything seems to fit, we become part of a whole, and that whole has meaning. Robert Byrd, a pragmatic explorer, spent months alone in the Arctic. Living in primitive conditions he became aware of the very fundamentals of existence. For Byrd the experience was an uplifting one.

> The day was dying, the night being born – but with great peace. Here were the imponderable processes and forces of

the cosmos, harmonious and soundless. Harmony, that was it! That was what came out of the silence – a gentle rhythm, the strain of a perfect chord, the music of the spheres perhaps. It was enough to catch that rhythm, momentarily to be myself a part of it. In that instant I could feel no doubt of man's oneness with the universe. The conviction came that that rhythm was too orderly, too harmonious, too perfect to be a product of blind chance – that, therefore, there must be purpose in the whole and not an accidental offshoot. It was a feeling that transcended reason, that went to the heart of man's despair and found it groundless. The universe was a cosmos, not a chaos; man was as rightfully a part of that cosmos as were the day and night.

Know Your Body

The Energy System

Whatever kind of work you perform, you must have energy to do it. The body is essentially a user of energy. All life-sustaining processes in the body use energy; if we can't produce energy we cannot live. Since any kind of exercise automatically requires the body to perform work, it follows that we must be able to generate enough energy, deliver it to where it is needed, and convert it into work once it has reached its destination.

The energy system is composed of several systems of the body: the respiratory system provides oxygen needed for the burning of the fuel; the cardiovascular system delivers the oxygen and fuel to the muscles; and energy conversion systems in the muscles convert the fuel and oxygen into muscular work or activity. There is in addition the complex digestive system, which of course provides the fuel, but its functioning processes are outside the scope of this book.

The respiratory system

The respiratory system is made up of two major components: the lungs, in which the gas exchange so vital for existence takes place, and the muscles of the chest wall, ribs, abdomen and the diaphragm. These muscles provide the pumping action which draws the air into the lungs and expels the carbon dioxide (CO_2) – a waste product – which the blood cells have exchanged for oxygen (O_2). The oxygen in the air we breathe is an essential element for the release of energy in the cells.

When we breathe in, air is drawn through the mouth and

nose which together act as filters, moisteners and warmers (though in exercise nearly 80 per cent of oxygen intake is through the mouth). It is then transported through increasingly smaller and smaller passages until it finally reaches the millions (nearly 600 million) of little air sacs or 'alveoli' which make up the lungs. The walls of these alveoli are so thin that it is possible for oxygen to diffuse directly through them and through the walls of the multitudes of capillaries surrounding the alveoli. There it is taken up by the haemoglobin in the blood cells in exchange for their cargo of CO_2 which then passes back out through the capillaries and alveoli from where it is expelled during breathing out. The actual surface space of these alveoli in the lungs of an average man would, if spread out, cover approximately half the surface of the centre court at Wimbledon!

Obviously, the more demands made by the body for energy, the greater the need for oxygen to convert fuel into work in the muscles. During rest about 350ml of oxygen leave the alveoli and about 200ml of CO_2 leave the blood every minute. During heavy exercise in a trained endurance athlete these figures can be increased up to 25 times. This increased capacity for gas exchange is a key element in an athlete's ability to improve performance.

There are two ways in which the lungs can respond to the body's increased demand for oxygen. They can pump faster or they can increase the volume of air which they pump with each breath. It is more efficient to increase the volume rather than the rate. While it is true that regular endurance training will increase the strength of the muscles which pump the lungs and therefore their ability to pump for longer and at a faster rate, the substantive change which most endurance athletes look for is an increase in the volume of air moved in and out at each respiration.

The average male has a total lung capacity of around 6 litres. If he were to breathe all the way out he would still have around 1.2 litres of air left in his lungs (his residual volume). The difference (4.8 litres) is what is known as his *vital capacity* which is usually 4–5 litres for men and 3–4 litres for women. However, it is not uncommon for endurance athletes to have vital capacities of 6–7 litres. One Olympic Gold Medallist cross-country skier had a vital capacity of 8.1 litres! *Potential* vital capacity is genetically determined but during adolescence it is possible to increase your vital capacity through training to its genetic limit. As an adult it is difficult to increase vital capacity much beyond the amount of potential you developed in your adolescence. In addition the strength of the respiratory muscles can be improved which contributes to both fuller utilization of one's vital capacity and an increased expulsion of air. Top endurance athletes can expel at least 80 per cent of the maximum functional capacity of their lungs in one second.

A combination of the above four factors – 1 genetic potential; 2 development of vital capacity; 3 strength of respiratory muscles; and 4 speed of expelling air, are the major factors which contribute to what is known as the *maximum minute ventilation*. Your maximum minute ventilation can be defined as the maximum quantity of air you can breathe in and out during one minute.

It is not often realized that another principal factor in high-level endurance exercise is not how much oxygen the athlete can *load* into his system but how much CO_2 he can *unload*. The threshold at which it is no longer possible to deliver oxygen to the body fast enough (or unload CO_2 fast enough) to maintain the release of energy in the cells is called the *anaerobic threshold*. Dr Robert Arnot, physician to a number of US national teams, explains that 'this training ability to unload excess CO_2 from the blood at high minute-volumes over a prolonged period is so important that it can be said to be the single most vital determinant for winning in endurance sports among athletes with similar constitutions.'

Hence Alberto Salazar in his world record, 2.08.13, 1981 marathon was able to maintain a minute ventilation of 140 litres of air per minute and Bill Koch, winner of the 1982 cross-country skiing World Cup, maintains a minute ventilation of 169 litres per minute over a 15 kilometre course.

The cardiovascular system

The heart, veins, arteries and capillaries make up the second major physical component of the Energy System. The heart pumps while the cardiovascular system carries the blood around the body. Together they could be called the energy delivery system. The blood can be thought of as the transport system for the oxygen from the lungs, the nutrients from the digestive

The Cardiovascular System

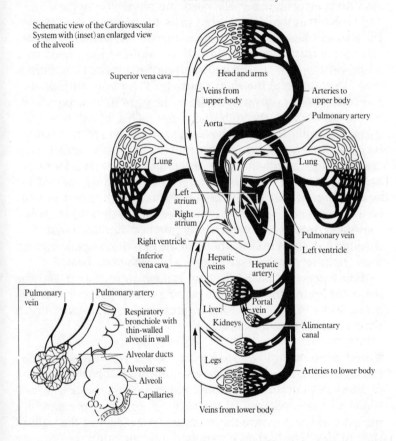

Schematic view of the Cardiovascular System with (inset) an enlarged view of the alveoli

Superior vena cava

Head and arms

Veins from upper body

Arteries to upper body

Aorta

Pulmonary artery

Lung

Lung

Left atrium

Right atrium

Pulmonary vein

Right ventricle

Left ventricle

Inferior vena cava

Hepatic veins

Hepatic artery

Portal vein

Liver

Kidneys

Alimentary canal

Legs

Arteries to lower body

Veins from lower body

Pulmonary vein

Pulmonary artery

Respiratory bronchiole with thin-walled alveoli in wall

Alveolar ducts

Alveolar sac

Alveoli

Capillaries

CO_2 O_2

system, glucose and glycogen from energy stores, hormones, glandular secretions, etc. It is also the main transport system for removing waste products from the tissues of the body, including CO_2. This ability of the heart to deliver promptly all the energy needed by the body cells and eliminate as quickly as possible the waste produced from the body's work is central to effective performance in all sports and physical activities.

The heart is usually referred to as a four-chambered pump. Each time it beats blood is being pumped from all four chambers simultaneously. On the right side, the right atrium, filled with blood returning from the body and carrying waste CO_2, pumps this blood down to the right ventricle. The right ventricle, full of blood previously pumped from the right atrium pumps its blood up to and through the lungs. This blood is carried through capillaries to the alveoli in the lungs where it exchanges its CO_2 for oxygen. It is the presence of high oxygen concentration in the blood which causes it to change its colour from blue to red. The blood is then returned to the left side of the heart where it collects in the left atrium. Each time the heart beats the oxygenated blood is pumped into the left ventricle and the blood in the left ventricle is pumped simultaneously out through the aorta into the body to the muscles, organs, etc. All four chambers of the heart empty with each heart beat.

This operation takes place 40 million times a year and the force generated from a year's beating could lift the owner 100 miles above the earth. Quite impressive for a muscular organ which weighs less than a pound!

Blood pressure   The blood from the left ventricle is pumped through the aorta into the arteries of the body. The arteries are a network of high pressure tubing which conduct the oxygen-rich blood to the capillaries of the body. Your blood pressure is a measure of the pressure this pumping exerts against the walls of the arteries. The higher, or *systolic*, figure measures the pressure at the high point of the heart contraction. The lower, or *diastolic*, figure measures the pressure against the arteries at the point where the heart relaxes and has stopped contracting. Average adult blood pressure figures are 120/80, systolic over diastolic.

The walls of arteries are made up of specialized muscles. They expand as your heart contracts in order to make room for the blood pumped into them from the heart. The arteries then contract so as to squeeze the blood further along and so assist the heart in its function. Through age, lack of exercise, stress and improper diet, arteries can lose their flexibility, or deposits of fat can build up on their inner walls (atherosclerosis) making it harder to pump the blood through them. The result is high blood pressure (as high as 250 systolic) creating excessive and chronic strain on the heart in particular. The possibility of heart failure or stroke grows with the rise in blood pressure. A regular programme of exercise (particularly aerobic) can in many cases reduce both systolic and diastolic blood pressure. (See Health, Fitness, and Well Being, pages 27–34.)

The blood from the arteries travels through ever smaller passages, arterioles and metarterioles until it finally reaches the tissue (e.g. muscle fibres) where it divides into capillaries which can be as dense as 2–3000 per square millimetre. It is in the capillaries that the O_2/CO_2 exchange takes place. After giving up their oxygen to the muscle cells and taking on the waste CO_2 byproduct from energy conversion, the blood cells travel further along the capillaries which slowly merge into the venules, and in turn into veins which ultimately lead back to the right atrium of the heart. Here the four-chambered pumping process of the heart is repeated until, with the return of the oxygenated blood to the heart, the cycle is completed.

Cardiac hypertrophy It has long been recognized that consistent exercise can result in some enlargement of the heart. Generally speaking sustained training in endurance sports like swimming, running and cycling, results in an increase in the *volume* of the left ventricle so that each stroke can push more blood out into the body. There is evidence that in strength and power sports like wrestling, weightlifting, etc., the *thickness* of the left ventricle wall is increased providing the extra power needed to pump blood through muscles which may be strongly contracted. So cardiac hypertrophy or 'athlete's heart' is very common and reflects the principle of specificity to the demands placed upon the body by the exercise performed. On the average, increases in heart volume in athletes over sedentary individuals is around 25 per cent.

It is important to lay to rest the scares concerning cardiac hypertrophy. Jean Corvisart (1755–1821), a French physician, first correlated enlarged hearts with certain diseases. But in 1879 Beneke, a German cardiologist, mistakenly concluded that an enlarged heart in athletes would lead to their premature death. Years later, in 1927, these claims led the Austrian doctors Deutsch and Kauf to pull their country's championship swimmers out of competition because their hearts were enlarged by 30–40 per cent. Nowadays it is commonly accepted that the hypertrophy of sportspeople's hearts is very different from the pathologically enlarged hearts studied by earlier physicians. In fact, increased volume and size of the heart can lead not only to improved performance but also to improved health.

The effect of training   During heavy exercise 60 per cent of the heart's output (which is determined by the heart rate and volume of blood pumped per beat) goes to the muscles of the body as opposed to only 4 per cent at rest. A normal heart during rest may pump 4 litres of blood a minute. The heart of a working marathoner may be pumping 30 litres of blood a minute. Great demand is placed upon the heart in physical performance and there are three ways, in addition to an increase in size (cardiac hypertrophy), by which a heart can meet this demand.

The best way to adapt to greater demand is to increase the volume of blood pumped. One way this can be achieved is by increasing the number of beats per minute, which is the normal response of the heart to higher demands and is something we all encounter when we begin to engage in any kind of aerobic training. But this is hard work for the heart; it is easier on the heart if we can increase its efficiency by reducing the number of beats per minute through increasing the volume of blood each single beat delivers to the arteries. This second adaptation is achieved through improved 'pre-loading' and reduced resistance or 'after-loading'. In 'pre-loading' the contracting muscles of the body actually squeeze more blood back into the heart through the veins. The heart is 'stretched' a little more to accommodate the extra volume of returning blood. Consequently there is more blood in the heart to be pumped out with each beat. In 'after-loading', since the training effect has produced lower blood pressure because the arteries are elastic and during exercise the capillaries dilate, there is reduced resistance to the blood being pumped from the heart. The left ventricle is emptied more fully with greater delivery on each beat and more space in the heart for the subsequent inflow. The combined effect of 'pre-loading' and 'after-loading' is an increase in the 'stroke volume' of each heart beat: a larger volume of blood is delivered with each beat. It is easy to see now why dehydration can be so deleterious in performance: less blood volume, thicker blood which is harder to pump, and consequently less blood delivered per beat. It is also clear why some top class athletes have gone in for blood doping: more blood in the body, larger volume of blood available from each beat, with the consequent delivery of more oxygen to the muscle cells. This process of 'pre-loading' and 'after-loading', as described by Arnot and Gaines in their book *Sports Selection*, is promulgated by them as a major contributor to athletic performance, particularly in endurance sports.

The third way in which the delivery of blood to the tissue is enhanced by training is through an increase in the heart's ability to do pressure work. This is particularly valuable for activities which require powerful muscle contraction like weight training, judo, riding, downhill skiing, etc. Sustained contraction in a muscle group compresses the arteries delivering blood. At 30–40 per cent of maximum contraction of a muscle it is no longer possible for the heart to push the blood through the capillaries in those muscles. Blood flow is stopped. Through training it is possible to increase the size of the heart muscle, particularly the septum wall and the walls of the left ventricle, which allows the heart to exert extra pressure and continue to deliver blood to muscle groups which are strongly contracted. It should be pointed out that while this extra size increases the ability of the heart to pump blood, it is not yet clear how substantially this will improve power performance nor that there are the same beneficial effects as there are in the increase in stroke volume.

VO$_2$Max This stands for the maximum oxygen uptake of the body, and is a key indicator of cardio-respiratory fitness. After years of trying to determine some fixed measure of the combined ability of the heart and lungs to deliver blood to the body, the measure of Maximum Oxygen Consumption has been accepted as the closest approximation of this joint function.

VO_2Max reflects not only the ability of the lungs to load oxygen and off-load CO_2, and the strength and volume of the heart strokes, but also the ability of the tissue and cells to accept the oxygen delivered to them and exchange the CO_2. It is a fairly comprehensive measure of how well you can be expected to perform in any endurance sport. It is also determined genetically: you can expect to increase your VO_2Max by no more than 20 per cent beyond genetically determined norm, no matter how hard you train. A major factor in your VO_2Max potential is the kinds of muscle fibres in your body (see The Power System, pages 72–81). In fact the changes that take place through training in the muscle cells, increasing their ability to metabolize fuel and oxygen, contribute *more* to your VO_2Max than improvement of the respiratory and cardiovascular systems. This is detailed in the sections on Strength (page 93) and Endurance (page 100).

But in addition to developing your full VO_2Max potential, a very well-trained athlete can sustain activity for extended periods of time at or near his anaerobic threshold: the point at which he is not able to deliver enough oxygen to the body to aerobically maintain the level at which energy is being expended. Sustained training over a number of years can result in the ability to perform sustained work at near the 90 per cent VO_2Max level and hence operate with a very high anaerobic threshold. This is rare but individuals like Alberto Salazar are said to be able to work at this high level of proficiency for long periods of time.

Fuel
The main sources of energy for the body are carbohydrates. The body stores carbohydrates as glycogen, which is subsequently broken up into glucose as needed, and as triglycerides, which are broken down into fatty acids and used as fuel like glucose. One gram of fat has twice the available energy of one gram of glucose (or protein, for that matter) hence its value as a long-term energy store. But its breakdown is slower. Glucose is the initial fuel for work and fats are the main form of stored fuel: a bit like kindling and logs in fire building. During energy metabolism in the cells, oxygen plays a key role in freeing the energy of the glucose and fat through a controlled oxidation or 'burning' of the fuel. The energy generated by this 'cellular

oxidation' is momentarily stored in what are known as High Energy Phospates: adenosine triphosphate (ATP) and creatine phosphate (CP). They carry the energy generated by the cellular oxidation of the glucose and fatty acids which is stored in a molecular bond holding the third phosphate molecule to the ATP. This energy is released at a biochemical level when needed for work. It is the first compound, ATP, which is most prominent in this process, CP being a back-up energy supply.

ATP   The energy of our fuels is not passed directly to the cells but rather is channelled through the energy-rich compound adenosine triphosphate (ATP). The energy carried by the ATP molecule is used for *all* energy requiring process in all cells. Muscular contraction, digestion, tissue repair, nerve transmission all use ATP. All members of the animal kingdom from the worm to humans use ATP in this way.

ATP releases its energy by joining with water in a process called hydrolisis which involves a very complex enzymatically controlled reaction with low temperature and minimum loss of energy. One of the three phosphate bonds is broken, releasing the stored energy to perform muscular work through biochemical processes. Left over from this reaction are adenosine diphosphate (ADP) plus an extra free phosphate molecule. Subsequently when you use oxygen to break down glucose or fatty acids and release their stored energy, this released energy is then used to put the free phosphate molecule back on to the ADP and so restore it as the energy-rich ATP, ready to release its phosphate molecule again to perform work in the cells. It's a bit like the big pile drivers which are burning fuel in their internal combustion engines so that they can repeatedly lift a heavy weight up so that it can be released again and again to fall and drive the pile into the ground.

The total amount of ATP in the body at any one time is enough to provide energy for maximal exercise for only 7–10 seconds! The process of breaking down carbohydrates to regenerate ATP is constant.

The energy systems

The phosphagen system (immediate energy)   It does not take any oxygen to utilize the ATP stored in the muscle cells. It is immediately available as a short-term source of energy. In

Energy Systems

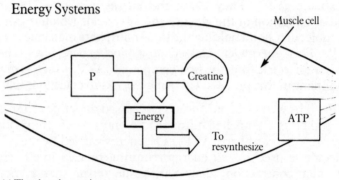

(a) The phosphocreatine system

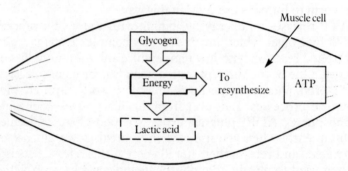

(b) The lactic acid system (anaerobic glycolysis)

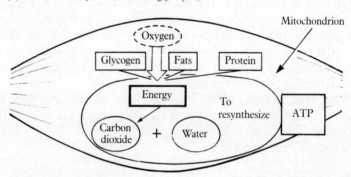

(c) The aerobic (oxygen) system

addition, CP is available to give up its phosphate molecule in order to restore ADP to ATP making it immediately available as an energy source again. If you were suddenly to realize that you had just ten minutes to reach the bank before closing time your phosphagen system will get you out of the door and on to the street. You won't be utilizing the energy from fats, glucose, etc. You are functioning on stored reserves of high energy phosphates. The 100-metre sprint, a tennis serve, or a tae kwon do kick all use this first stage energy system. It is the energy immediately available for short term actions, be they slow or quick, gentle or explosive. The phosphagen system takes very few enzymes to convert the stored energy into work so the steps for making it available are brief. It does not rely upon any immediate source of oxygen or stored fuel. It is there, in your cells, immediately available, now. There is enough stored phosphate energy to walk briskly for about one minute, run the beginning of a marathon for 20–30 seconds or perform an all-out exertion for 6–7 seconds.

The lactic acid system or anaerobic glycolisis (short-term energy) This immediate energy of the phosphagen system will be depleted unless ATP regeneration begins. You will run out of energy fast which is what happens near the end of a sprint or a series of repetitions in weight training. When this happens, the second state of energy generation, anaerobic glycolysis or the lactic acid system, takes over. If your phosphagen system will get you out of the door on your way to the bank, the lactic acid system will be your main energy source during the 5-minute run to the bank itself. Since you must continue to generate ATP to do work, once the immediate stores are used up, you will begin to generate ATP as quickly as possible from available glucose sources. The breakdown of glucose – glycolysis – is most efficient if it involves oxygen. However, it is possible to break glucose down, partially releasing some of its energy, without the use of oxygen. This process, anaerobic glycolysis, does allow your body to resynthesize ATP rapidly. But it only provides one third of the energy possible from full aerobic glycolysis and, more problematically, it leaves a by-product from the incomplete breakdown in the muscle cells. This by-product, *lactic acid*, accumulates in the muscle cells and if not broken down completely will eventually build up to the point where it interrupts the continuing functioning of the muscle cells: fatigue sets in. And with the fatigue comes pain.

In a sense, the lactic acid system is buying time. It takes on the job of maintaining the ATP supply until a more long-term measure can sustain the production of the ATP.

The aerobic system (long-term energy) The aerobic system of energy production is the most efficient and substantial of the three systems which operate in the body. If you are going to engage in any sustained activity for more than 5 or 6 minutes, it comes into play. Let's say that the branch of the bank you go to has a huge queue so you continue your run to the next branch, 10 minutes down the road. All the effects of the deep breathing you have been doing up to this point will now begin to filter down to the actual biochemical level of energy conversion. The aerobic system takes over. Aerobic exercise is simply exercise which engages you in the aerobic production of energy. Marathon running, cross-country skiing, swimming, cycling, walking are all fundamentally aerobic exercises. After 6–10 minutes your increased oxygen uptake will provide all the oxygen you need to break down the glucose completely, both increasing the amount of energy produced from the fuels and decreasing the lactic acid build-up and its accompanying muscle fatigue.

General characteristics of the energy systems

Phosphagen (ATP-PC) System	Lactic Acid System	Aerobic (Oxygen)
Anaerobic	Anaerobic	Aerobic
Very rapid	Rapid	Slow
Chemical fuel: PC	Food fuel: glycogen	Food fuels: glycogen, fats, and protein
Very limited ATP production	Limited ATP production	Unlimited ATP production
Muscular stores limited	By-product, lactic acid, causes muscular fatigue	No fatiguing by-products
Used with sprint or any high-power short-duration activity	Used with activities of 1 to 3 min duration	Used with endurance long-duration activities

Source: Edward L. Fox, *Sports Physiology*, 2nd edn, Holt Saunders International Editions, 1984, p. 22.

According to Eric Newsholme of Oxford University, our fat burning mechanism comes into play after about 30 minutes of sustained exercise. Prior to that you are running on glycogen, the body's immediate energy stores (or primary boosters, used in instant effort, like climbing stairs or lifting weights). Glycogen must be replaced quickly – hence the thirst and hunger pangs experienced after short bursts of intense activity. Counter to this most exercisers report feeling no hunger after longer bouts of activity (understandable since the digestive system gets 'parked' for a while during sustained effort).

Theoretically the only limit to how long you can engage in aerobic activity is the stores of fuel in your body. Practically there are other metabolic and biochemical constraints. Still, a sustained rate of five minutes a mile over a 26-mile marathon is no mean accomplishment and the more prodigious efforts of triathletes speak even more emphatically of the potential of the human body.

If we return to the respiratory and cardiovascular systems and their combined measurement, VO_2Max, we can now see that our VO_2Max is the measurement of our maximal capacity for the aerobic synthesis of energy. And since this measurement also indicates how much work we can produce without going over our anaerobic threshold and shifting back to anaerobic glycolysis, it should become clear that the training effect on our heart and lungs increases our ability to function at the top end of our potential in aerobic exercise. Improving our respiratory functioning through enhancing its vital capacity and its minute volume work will allow us to off-load the greatest amount of the by-product CO_2 and load the blood with the necessary oxygen for aerobic glycolysis. Training our cardiovascular capacity particularly through increasing our heart's stroke volume and improving its pre-loading and after-loading abilities will enhance the amount of oxygen-laden blood available to the cells. These factors, combined with the equally important physiological changes which take place in the muscle fibres themselves (see Endurance, pages 100–10), produce a capacity for a high level of sustained endurance work.

The Power System

Human beings are made for movement. Without movement life as we know it would not exist. All systems of exercise require movement and all have the basic movement principles in common. We move ourselves by contracting our skeletal muscles. The skeletal muscles move our bony levers in relation to each other and the result is movement in space. Put simply, the power system of the body consists of muscles which are attached to the bones of the skeleton by means of tendons, a connective tissue, and joints (articulations) which are usually reinforced structurally with another connective tissue called a ligament.

Skeleton
The skeleton is the bony framework of the body. A complex system of levers, it conforms to the basic laws of physics. The use of the levers increases the efficiency of the contractile work of the muscles. A lever system always consists of a lever (in this case the bone); a fulcrum (the joint); resistance (the weight of the body or object being moved); and the effort (the action of the muscle).

There are different classes of levers and they perform different jobs in different parts of the body. In the illustration the three classes of levers and representative instances in the body are given.

In the case of the first class lever, the most amount of work is accomplished with the least effort. It is the most efficient lever system, but its range of movement tends to be more limited. Lifting the head to look upwards involves this first class system. It is very stable and quite powerful but the actual movement of the head is limited.

A second class lever is not as efficient as the previous system, but it has the advantage of being able to have both the resistance (i.e. the weight of the body) and the effort (muscle contraction) on the same side of the fulcrum. This makes pivoting on the ball of the foot possible.

Third class levers are the least efficient. However, because the resistance is away from the fulcrum (joint) and the effort (muscle), it is possible to move objects at quite a distance from

The Mechanics of Movement

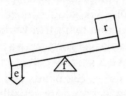
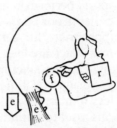

1st class lever. The fulcrum (joint) always lies between the effort (muscle) and the resistance (weight). This is the most efficient class of lever. With a constant weight, the longer the distance f–e, relative to the distance f–r, the less muscle effort required.
f = fulcrum △ ; e = effort ◊; r = resistance □

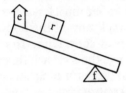
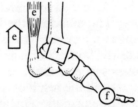

2nd class lever. The resistance always lies between the fulcrum (joint) and the effort (muscle), such as when pushing/lifting a wheelbarrow. In this case, the longer f–e distance relative to the shorter f–r distance provides a good mechanical advantage for the muscle lifting the body weight onto the heads of the metatarsals.

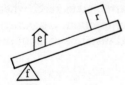
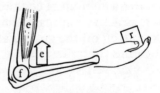

3rd class lever. The muscular effort is placed between the weight and the joint, providing the least efficient mechanical advantage. To compare 3rd and 2nd class levers: lifting a 50 lb box with your arms takes significantly more muscle effort than lifting your 150 lb body by standing on the heads of your metatarsals.

the source of effort and the fulcrum point, as in curling a barbell or swinging a tennis racquet.

Skeletal size and proportion are important factors in determining sports performance. While we will all have the same number of bones in our body (208), certain proportional lengths are more appropriate for certain sports. A good runner will often have legs which are long in proportion to his trunk whereas a good cross-country skier may have a larger torso with a large chest cavity. Sprinters will usually have a narrow pelvis which allows the legs a more direct line to follow. Big hands and feet are an obvious asset to swimmers. Knock-knees are actually an asset for alpine skiers!

Muscles

Muscles do only two things: they contract or they stop contracting, i.e. relax. A muscle does not 'lengthen' or stretch itself, it is lengthened or stretched by other muscles or perhaps by gravity. The muscle is the basic work unit of the body. All movement is the result of some form of contracting from the muscles of the body. The heart beating, the stomach digesting or the pupils contracting, as well as legs running and arms swinging, are all the result of muscle contractions.

When speaking of movement, there are three types of muscle contractions. The first, *concentric*, takes place when the muscle is active and shortening, e.g. performing a chin-up on a bar over your head. The second, *excentric*, takes place when the muscle is active but being lengthened, e.g. lowering yourself back to the floor after a chin-up. The third, *isometric*, takes place when the muscle is active but maintaining a contraction, e.g. when you hold yourself off the ground at a fixed distance without raising or lowering yourself.

Muscle types

There are three kinds of muscle:

The first type are the smooth, non-striated muscles. These make up the blood vessels and the walls of the hollow visceral organs like the stomach and intestines. They are controlled by the autonomic nervous system and hence not under our direct conscious control; they are regulated by the general needs and conditions of the body (see The Control System, pages 81–92).

The second type of muscle is the cardiac muscle, which consists of specialized muscle cells found only in the heart. Because of a special relationship with the nerves which innervate the cardiac muscle it contracts rhythmically and automatically without the need for direct stimulation from the central nervous system and will do so for the life of the individual.

The third type of muscle is the striated muscle or skeletal muscle. These are the power force for all movement of the body through space. The skeleton and its lever system is moved by striated muscles. This type of muscle, which makes up the bulk of the muscle of the body (more than 430 of them) is controlled by the voluntary nervous system. In most cases we can choose to move these muscles in order to perform the myriad movements required by daily life and exercise.

It is these striated, skeletal muscles which concern us most in movement, and the rest of this section is concerned with their function. Muscles are connected to bones by *tendons* (bone to bone connections are called *ligaments*). The tendon is a connective tissue which does not itself contract. It is more or less elastic

The Structure of Skeletal Muscle

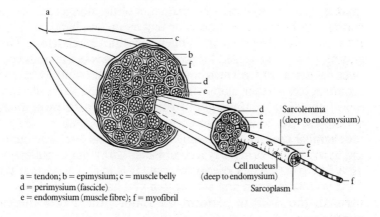

a = tendon; b = epimysium; c = muscle belly
d = perimysium (fascicle)
e = endomysium (muscle fibre); f = myofibril

and its elastic properties are very important when working with flexibility and stretching. The tendon merges at its attachment to the bone with the tough protective covering of the bone, the *periostium*. At the muscle end it merges with the protective sheath of connective tissue which surrounds the muscle, the *epimysium*. Both the periostium and epimysium are connective tissues, like the tendon.

Structurally the striated muscle can be thought of as a little like the Russian wooden dolls: each time you take off a layer you find another one inside. Each muscle is made up of a number of fasciculi, or *muscle bundles*, each bundle wrapped by a layer of connective tissue called *perimysium*. Each bundle is in turn made up of a collection of *muscle fibres* surrounded by connective tissue called *endomysium*. The muscle fibres are the work unit and are in turn made up of a collection of *myofibrils*. It is within these myofibrils that the actual contracting process takes place in the muscle.

In each myofibril are a number of *sacromere*, stacked end to end like carriages of a train. Each sacromere can shorten in length a little and as they do so the myofibril itself shortens. All the myofibrils in a muscle fibre (or cell) contract in unison. When you bend your arm at half strength half the muscle fibres will be mobilized, but each will work at 100 per cent effort (rather than all the muscle fibres working at half steam).

Each sacromere is made up of two basic proteins: actin and myosin. Actin and myosin filaments slide along each other similar to the way in which your fingers on one hand can slide into the space between the fingers on your other hand. This sliding process is caused by molecular bridges being built connecting actin and myosin and then being broken down and reconnected further along the line drawing the actin filament along the line of the myosin filament. As with most body processes, the muscle contraction at this stage stops being a mechanical process and becomes a biochemical one. The building of molecular bridges is accomplished through the utilization of ATP, your body's energy supply. It is at this level that the food you have eaten and the oxygen you have breathed is used through the ATP to perform the simple function of muscle contraction.

Muscle fibre types

To meet the wide-ranging demands of different activities – fast or slow, strong or gentle, short bursts or constant activity – we have different kinds of muscle fibres. All are generated through combinations of three main muscle fibre types: Slow Twitch (ST) and Fast Twitch (FT) and an intermediate type known as Fast Twitch A (FTA), which will be discussed later.

FT fibres contract very quickly, three times as fast as ST fibres, and very forcefully, up to ten times more powerfully than ST fibres. They are controlled by large motor nerves which conduct messages very rapidly to and from the central nervous system. FT fibres have a large diameter and can be increased in size by appropriate training (see pages 78–79). While they generate energy very quickly, their rapid utilization of the stored muscle glycogen is usually at the expense of incomplete glucose break-down and resultant build-up of lactic acid. This means that FT fibres, which rely primarily on anaerobic metabolism for energy are good for strong short bursts but suffer from rapid exhaustion. Sprinting, a boxing punch, a karate kick, a high jump, a ballet leap . . . all these use FT fibres.

ST fibres are designed for sustained work. Marathon runners use ST fibres almost exclusively. They operate aerobically and break down glucose completely. This, as we have seen, results in less lactic acid build-up and hence the reduction or postpone-ment of fatigue and pain. In order to do this, ST fibres have a much larger number of *mitochondria* than FT fibres (up to 12 times more). Mitochondria are the powerhouses of the muscle cells and help convert glucose into energy (ATP) aerobically. ST fibres also have larger stores of *myoglobin* (up to 3 times more than FT fibres), a substance similar to haemoglobin, the oxygen carrier in the red blood cells. Myoglobin works in conjunction with the mitochondria to ensure a constant supply of oxygen for the aerobic production of energy. On top of this, ST fibres have an increased vascularization: they have more arteries, capillaries and veins than FT fibres and hence greater oxygen supply. Distance running, swimming, cross-country skiing, all rely on ST fibres to do the work.

The next time you eat chicken, notice the difference of the colour of the meat. The leg meat will be darker in colour: it is made up mostly of ST fibre full of mitochondria and myoglobin and employed in sustained walking. The breast and wings are lighter as this muscle, made up of FT fibre, is used only for occasional short explosive bursts of activity.

So whereas FT fibres use quick, immediate glucose, which they only break down partially, ST fibres use not only glucose but also stored energy deposits: fat. As you run, cycle or swim for more than 30 minutes, you begin to use a larger and larger percentage of fat as your ST fibres draw on that source of energy for sustained work. So not only are ST fibres more efficient in converting glucose, they are also the major burners of stored fat deposit.

To lose weight through exercise it is necessary to perform sustained, aerobic activity at a constant level so that the energy stored in fat can be tapped by the ST fibres in your body.

There is a third type of fibre which seems to be like an FT fibre type but has certain ST characteristics and can adapt through training towards either FT or ST properties, as power or endurance demands are made upon it.

All sports require varying degrees of ST and FT fibres. While a tennis serve is obviously an explosive, FT function, and a marathon run requires the sustained energy of the ST fibre, most sports require a mixture of the two activities. A soccer player must be able to sustain repeated runs up and down the field throughout a 45-minute half, and yet be able to produce an explosive shot on goal when required. A cross-country skier needs sustained energy to complete the course but powerful thrusts with his poling arms and shoulders require strong fast movements.

Training effects on slow and fast twitch muscle fibres

While you cannot change your genetic makeup and hence the proportion of ST and FT fibres in your muscles, you can train your muscle fibres to work more efficiently at what they are designed to do. Through endurance training you improve more than just your level of cardiovascular fitness. You improve the capacity of the ST fibres to utilize their energy sources – glucose, fat and oxygen – more effectively. Mitochondria increase in number and size. The enzymes necessary to facilitate the whole process are increased. Myoglobin is increased by up to 80 per cent, allowing more oxygen to be available in the ST fibres at any given time. The ups and downs of oxygen demand are thus smoothed, reducing the likelihood of having to resort to anaerobic, fatigue producing energy systems. The muscle cells also speed up their ability to mobilize their stored reserves of glycogen and fat. Many exercise physiologists maintain that the main factor in improved endurance performance is not due to improved cardiovascular and respiratory performance but rather to muscle physiology adaptation to training.

In FT fibres, the most noticeable training change is in the increase in size. Muscle hypertrophy (increase in size) is substantial in FT fibres, particularly during strength training. (The evidence is less consistent concerning the hypertrophy of ST fibres.) You cannot increase the *number* of muscle fibres, only their size. This increase results in more power. Stored reserves of high energy phosphagens are increased in FT fibres through strength training. These increase tolerance to lactic acid build-up, which means that FT fibres can function for longer periods of time with lactic acid present before fatigue sets in.

As mentioned before, the intermediate (FTA) fibres adapt towards the type of training demands which you make upon them. If you engage in strength training they increase in size and stored glycogen reserves. If you practise endurance training, they increase in mitochondria and myoglobin content and in aerobic metabolism of the energy source.

Other factors determining power

There are other factors which determine the power and speed of a muscle's movement. One factor is the relationship of a muscle's size or, more precisely, cross-sectional area, to its length. The wider the muscle is across the middle, the more powerful the force it can exert – the quadraceps in your thigh is going to be stronger than the biceps in your arm. And, through strength training which results in an increase of the cross-sectional area of your biceps, you will experience a resultant increase in strength of your arm.

One way of establishing the relationship between the power of a movement and the speed at which it can be performed is through establishing the force velocity curve for a given muscle group. If you were to lift a heavy barbell you would do so at a much slower speed than you would a very light barbell. In between these two extremes is a wide range of possible speed and strength relationships. The force velocity curve for each muscle or muscle group reflects both the relative combination of FT and ST fibres in a muscle group as well as the training influences on its performance (see graph for example of this when cycling at 110 rpm).

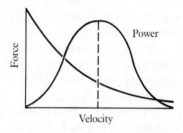

It is the combination of all these factors – muscle fibre types, muscle cross-sectional area, the training effects of endurance or strength on muscle makeup, stored reserves of energy, connective tissue elasticity and finally muscle temperature – which will determine the power, speed, contractile strength and endurance capacity of a given muscle group.

A change of 5 degrees centigrade in the actual temperature of a muscle will increase its performance by up to 50 per cent, and a muscle's elasticity can be enhanced through proper training and stretching techniques. Whether you are dancing to *Swan Lake*, throwing a judo opponent, rowing down the Thames or simply taking a walk through the countryside, the above factors all influence your performance.

Heredity Heredity and training are the two parameters which determine your individual control over the above factors. You can't change your heredity but you can cultivate the physical potential you were born with. Considerable variations in the proportions of FT and ST fibres in a given muscle group are to be found from individual to individual. These proportions are fixed at birth, hence sayings such as 'a sprinter is born not made'. This variation in muscle fibres explains why an elite athlete might excel in one sport and be quite unremarkable in a sport requiring a different ratio of FT and ST fibres. Sprinters don't make good marathon runners.

But these genetic determinants need not keep us from performing a chosen sport well until we begin to enter the higher levels of competition. For the Zola Budds, Arnold Schwarzeneggers, and John McEnroes, these hereditary factors are make or break conditions for success. For most of us they simply contribute more or less to our relative degree of accomplishment. If you are seriously interested in competing in a sport, martial art, dance competition, then by all means set your goals in the light of the crucial factors which will influence your success.

Whatever your sport, you can improve your performance through improving the functioning of your power system. Determine the general physiological demands which your sport places on you and the specific demands it places on different muscle groups in your body. Then establish training routines, in accordance with expert advice, to cultivate these potentials within the power system of your body.

The Control System

The control system is the most sophisticated and complex of the three main body systems. It is easy to question the need to know about synapses, reflex arcs, the sympathetic nervous system and other similar components of the control system. Yet any tennis player who has hit the ball out of play for the hundredth time as they rush the net has got to know how to interrupt bad habits. Anyone who suffers from over-anxiety before a competition, or stage-fright before a performance, must be interested in controlling the over-arousal of his sympathetic nervous system. Any practitioner of martial arts who has reflexively tried to catch herself in a fall rather than rolling with it will want to know how to cope with her reflex arcs. Any dancer trying to learn a new skill will want to know how fine motor skills are differentiated in the premotor cortex and how the newly-learned ability is stored in the motor cortex, cerebellum and spine. And anyone making special demands upon his or her body will want to be aware of the variety of messages and signals from the proprioceptive nerves, and how they can help improve performance through accurate feedback. The control system is not just a complex network of neurons, axons and dendrites – it is your vital system of listening to what your body has to say to you and then communicating what you want it to do for you. It is your trusted messenger, your information gatherer and your most intimate confidant. Remember, every square millimetre of your body is permeated with your control system. In fact you might even say that the only real purpose of your power and energy systems is to carry around and sustain your control system!

The purpose of the control system as a whole is remarkably straightforward. It collects information via its sensory nerves and pools it all in the central nervous system where it is filed, collated and interpreted. It then makes decisions about how it wants to respond to the input and sends these decisions back out to the body via the motor nerves where they are put into action.

Central nervous system (CNS): *organization*

The central nervous system is the most complex system in the entire human being. It consists of the brain and the spinal cord and acts as a control centre for all the information our body receives and transmits through its network of nerves. Every function in our body seems to be double, triple, quadrupally checked and counter-checked by it. No movement takes place without several levels of control entering into play.

The brain is divided into three parts: the forebrain, the midbrain and the hindbrain (see chart opposite). These divisions are for convenience sake and each of the three parts has a multitude of functions, but when learning and performing sports skills or any of the structured skills required by dance, martial arts, yoga, etc. listed in the second half of this book, there are several subdivisions of these three sections of the brain which play a central role.

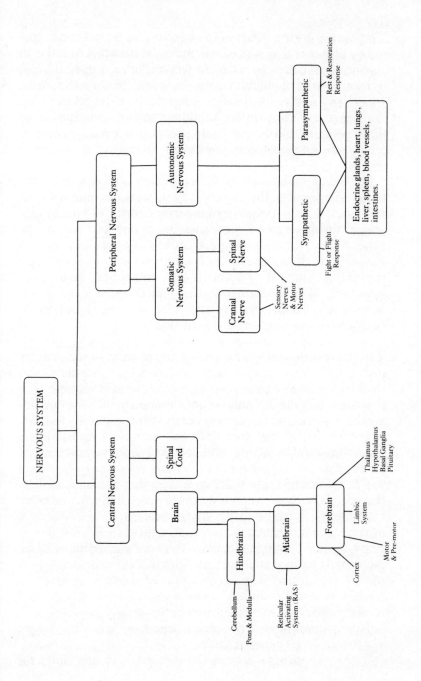

The forebrain

The motor cortex   Part of the forebrain or frontal cortex, the motor cortex is that part of the human brain which is active in learning movement patterns. In fact it is often termed the *skill learning area* of the brain. Just as the frontal cortex is the area in which we think and generalize abstractedly, so too when we are involved in cognitively thinking about movement, or differentiating and discriminating between one muscle group or another in relationship to movement, we are using our motor cortex.

In the beginning stages of learning a new skill, this area of the brain will organize the movements, in particular fine and delicate ones. The messages from the motor cortex will travel via a major 'throughway' of the brain, the pyramidal tract, to the lower motor nerves in the spinal cord from where they are then passed on to the muscles of the body to perform movements like untying a knot or learning a new movement in a dance sequence. When we are analysing and thinking about movement and sensation we are probably working in our motor cortex to understand and learn the skill.

The premotor area   This area, lying in front of the primary motor area, helps organize larger and more complete movement patterns, such as a tennis serve or the crawl in swimming. The premotor area doesn't analyse or discriminate. We draw on this area of our brain when carrying out movements already learned. It is often called the *sports skills area* because it seems to be a focus of control for all the skills and techniques we have learned about which we no longer have to think consciously. So, when you are learning a new skill, say a drop shot in tennis, initially the specific area of the motor cortex which controls voluntary movements in those body parts involved in the skill will organize the movement as you experiment and explore different grips, swings, footings, etc. Once you have learned the skill, the movement pattern no longer needs to be held so consciously in the motor cortex. The organization of the now generalized movement can be shifted to the premotor area. Rather than *thinking* about the movement you automatically *coordinate* it. It becomes a part of your movement repertoire to be drawn upon as needed. *It has become a skill.*

The relationship between the motor cortex and premotor

cortex is one of constant shuttling back and forth depending upon how much you are learning a new technique and how much you are calling upon an already acquired skill.

The midbrain

The reticular activating system (RAS) By comparison the midbrain is small and seems to be a corridor for messages from the forebrain and hindbrain to travel back and forth via a complex web of nerves called the Reticular Activating System (RAS). Arousal, or activation, is a neurophysiological process which seems to be regulated or transmitted by the RAS. It operates a bit like the dimmer switch which allows you to control not only the on/off of the 'current' flow to your brain but also gradually to increase or decrease the amount of stimulation flowing in it.

The hindbrain

The cerebellum While both the motor and premotor areas are involved in learning skills and initiating voluntary movement, they rely heavily upon the cerebellum, located at the base of the skull, to help coordinate the actions of large groups of muscles. The cerebellum is important in providing the unconscious smoothing out of movements and the integration of one movement with the next. The cerebellum is also the 'clearing house' for information coming from the proprioceptive nerves which convey information about pressure, balance, tension, speed of movement and so on.

It is convenient to say that movement is 'volitionally' controlled in the premotor cortex, but in fact the organizations and control of a movement is thought to be laid down as a pattern, or engram, which is stored not only in the motor cortex and premotor cortex but also in the cerebellum, basal ganglia (another part of the forebrain) and spine. Together they all orchestrate a smooth, constantly regulated flow of movement. And most of the process is unconscious.

The nerves: *the messenger boys*

The Nerves – 'the telephone cables'   All messages within the body travel via neurons, more commonly known as nerves. There are three kinds of nerves: *afferent* or *sensory nerves* carry information from the periphery of the body to the CNS; *efferent* or *motor nerves* carry information and instructions from the CNS to the muscles, as well as some glands and organs. *interneurons*, as the name implies, connect one nerve with another. Often they connect a motor nerve with a sensory nerve, but in the brain interneurons often connect to other interneurons.

All nerves are composed of three major elements. The first is the *cell body*, which is the control centre of the nerve, with its nucleus and genetic code. The *axon* carries messages away from the cell body of the nerve. If it is part of a sensory nerve, then the axon will be taking a message from the periphery and carrying it towards the centre to be processed in the CNS. If it is a motor nerve, it will be carrying the message from the CNS towards the periphery to tell a muscle to do something. The *dendrites* are multitudes of information-collecting fibres leading into the cell body. If part of a sensory nerve, the dendrites might collect information on heat, pressure, muscle tension, etc. and take it to the cell body where it is organized to be sent on through the axon to the CNS. In a motor nerve, the dendrites collect signals from other nerves in the CNS. The messages are then sent out via the axon to the muscle cells to stimulate them into action.

The synapse – 'bridging the gap'   As messages are relayed from one nerve to the next, they must travel across a gap or space called a *synapse*. While the message is transmitted 'electrically' within a nerve and along its axon (hence the very quick speed of nervous messages), the transfer of signals from one nerve to the next is done chemically. Just as in the power system, where at the cell level the process of muscular contraction takes place biochemically between the actin and myosin proteins in the sacromere, so too, at this stage of transmission, the message is passed biochemically from nerve to nerve.

The peripheral nervous system (PNS): *self-regulation*

The somatic nervous system (SNS): collection and action
The somatic nervous system is concerned with the transmission
and reception of information between the body and the central
nervous system. It is the vehicle for conscious and voluntary
control of the body as well as reflexes. It is categorized into
twelve cranial and 31 spinal nerves. But it can be thought of
simply as all the nerves outside the brain and spine which are
involved in organizing movement. They are divided into two
categories: sensory and motor.

The Sensory Nerves *The exteroceptors* – collecting information
from outside the body. In order to be able to function in any
manner at all we must have constant sensory input. In fact we
are receiving thousands of discreet pieces of information every
second which have to be sorted out by the CNS. The various
sensory systems which collect this information from the outside are called exteroceptors since they receive information
from *external* stimulation. Sight, hearing, smell and heat sensitivity are examples of these. You use your eyes to watch an
approaching football so as to gauge when to strike. You use your
ears to listen to where your opponent is behind you on a squash
court or to the sound of your skis as they travel over the snow in
order to gauge how fast you are travelling.

The proprioceptors – collecting information from inside the
body.   There are, as well, other kinds of sensory nerves – the
proprioceptors (or *interoceptors*) through which the body gains
precise and accurate information about its balance, alignment,
positioning and sense of movement. Our inner ear, for example,
is a proprioceptor and is not actually used for hearing external
sounds but rather to help us determine which direction is 'up',
whether we are turning in a pirouette or flying through the air in
an aikido fall. (A gyroscope serves a similar function in helping
the pilot of a plane to gauge where up and down is.) Another
example of proprioceptors are the pressure receptors located
throughout the body but found most densely in the palm and
fingers of the hand and the soles of the feet. They tell us how

tightly we are gripping the handle of our tennis racquet or help us gauge precisely the amount of weight on the ball of our foot if we are maintaining a balance in yoga or a ballet class. Through them we can adjust to minute changes of balance. There are also *position receptors* in the muscles which help us determine how much a muscle has been lengthened and how rapidly it is contracting, in the tendons where they give stronger and stronger signals as the tendon is stretched thereby guarding against over-stretching, and in the joints where they tell us when the joint has neared the end of its range of movement. All together proprioceptors give the CNS precise information about *where the body is in relationship to itself.*

As an example, close your eyes, extend your arms out to the side and now slowly bring your hands together in front of you to touch your index fingers without watching. How close did you come? Maybe within an inch, or less? You know where the two hands are in relationship to each other through your proprioceptors. In conjunction with the exteroceptors, the proprioceptors are crucial for any kind of skill learning and self-adjustment as you perform the simplest of t'ai-chi forms, stand on your head in yoga or race down a ski slope.

The motor nerves *The motor units* – putting it all into action. While the various exteroceptors and proprioceptors collect information, the motor units could be said to move the muscles. Muscles are made up of thousands of muscle fibres and each of these is innervated by a single terminal branch of a motor nerve. Each motor nerve, however, may innervate a number of muscle fibres, the number depending on the degree of control required of a particular muscle group. All the muscle fibres controlled by one motor nerve are called a *motor unit*. A motor unit in a muscle controlling an eye movement may only have 10 muscle fibres in it whereas a motor unit in your hamstrings may have 8,000 muscle fibres. No matter how many muscle fibres a motor unit controls two things are constant. When a motor nerve fires, all of the muscle fibres it controls will contract, be they 10 or 10,000. There is no such thing as only part of a motor unit contracting. Secondly, there is no such thing as a weak or strong contracting motor unit. It is an all or nothing principle. This means that in order for the CNS to increase the force of a muscle's contractions, it will have to increase the *number* of motor units brought into play and increase the *frequency* of the firing of the motor units so that they continue to contract. However, not all motor units in a muscle fire at the same time. In fact, it is essential that they don't, otherwise it would be almost impossible to control the contractions.

Motor units are comprised of either all Fast Twitch, all Slow Twitch, or all Intermediate fibres. *Fast Twitch* motor units are engaged for power work and *Slow Twitch* motor units are used for endurance work. As mentioned before, motor units don't all fire at once. It really depends upon the kind of task required of them. While it is generally true, for example, that one of the physiological factors which contributes to a weightlifter's ability to perform is the *synchronous* firing pattern of his motor units (i.e. many motor units in his muscles all being required simultaneously), it is equally true that a good cyclist or cross-country skier will develop an *asynchronous* firing pattern in his motor units (some motor units will be firing while others are resting) to preserve strength and stamina. Most of our daily activities and most exercise use primarily asynchronous firing patterns.

Reflexes: the reflex arc – The simplest picture. Your doctor tapping just below your knee with his rubber hammer sets off a reflex known as a Gamma Reflex Loop. A sensory nerve carries a message from the muscle to spine and a motor nerve returns a command from spine to muscle: the hammer hits, the knee jerks. Dozens of 'automatic' reflexes like this (though many are more sophisticated and involve the cerebellum and even the cortex) are essential for the smooth, coordinated and automatic functioning of the body. They enable us, for instance, to place our feet correctly, to maintain balance or to keep our head level. So although we cannot 'exercise' or 'strengthen', or most often even 'control' these reflexes, a basic understanding of what they are telling us and how they influence our performance can be invaluable. The section on flexibility illustrates how a knowledge of the myotactic reflexes will help us to increase flexibility safely. Understanding some of the head-righting reflexes helps us develop appropriate posture and alignment in dance or golf. The startle reflex interferes with learning basic falling techniques in aikido and other martial arts and is a part of general stress producing behaviours. Learning a new form of movement often involves unlearning deep-seated patterns of movement and in many cases learning to inhibit reflexive responses. No wonder it takes such a long time, concerted attention and systematic retraining of the nervous system to perfect our skills and techniques!

Stretch Reflex

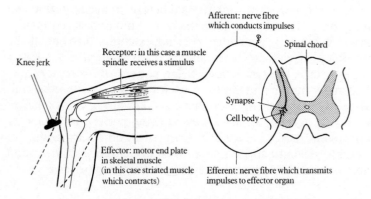

When the tendon is sharply tapped the muscle is stretched. (N.B. The stimulus is by stretching of the muscle spindle.) Nerve messages pass into the spinal chord and out to the muscle which then contracts.

Autonomic nervous system (ANS): maintaining the internal environment

The autonomic nervous system parallels the spinal cord and is concerned with maintaining a stable and consistent *internal* environment. In addition to our responses to the environment, we are being constantly informed about what is happening inside our body during each movement. Whether we are competing for our black belt in judo, practising a meditation technique, digesting our dinner or watching a horror film on television, our ANS is regulating our internal functions to ensure that they are in accord with the needs that our environment and current activity require from our body. Your heart rate increases in preparation for the judo competition, your stomach growls at the prospect of a good meal, your pulse rate goes down in meditation or your pupils dilate at the sight of the bushes rustling prior to the werewolf emerging on the television screen. These functions are all directly influenced or controlled by your ANS.

The ANS is divided into two halves: the sympathetic and the parasympathetic. They tend to operate as opposing pairs:

Sympathetic (Fight or Flight Response)	*Parasympathetic (Rest and Restoration Response)*
Pupils in eyes dilate, open wide	Pupils constrict, eyes accommodate for closer vision
Capillaries in muscles dilate, blood flows to muscles more easily	Capillaries in muscles contract, blood returns to central organs
Heart rate quickens	Heart rate slows
Stomach muscles relax, stop working	Gastric juices secreted
Adrenal glands and liver: secretion of adrenalin and mobilization of liver glycogen	Stomach, gall bladder, small intestine walls: peristaltic action, emptying passing food and digested substances along digestive chain
Intestines and colon: relax, stop working	Rectum and urinary sphincters relaxing, emptying

From this it can be seen that when we are engaged in strenuous physical activity the sympathetic system is operating to ensure that the internal functions of our body are being mobilized to meet the demands of activity: blood is pumped at an increased rate and directed to the skeletal muscles; adrenalin, the primary stimulant of physical activity, is secreted; digestion stops, breathing rate increases; pupils open wide for information gathering. When physical arousal ceases the parasympathetic system comes into play: the body's skeletal muscles work less; blood is directed to the digestive organs so that food digestion and assimilation can take place; the heartbeat slows; breathing is easier; waste products can be emptied from the colon; in the longer term the process of rest and restoration can take place. It may *seem* that nothing is happening during parasympathetic arousal but this could not be further from the truth!

The Autonomic Nervous System directly influences our performance at all levels of physical activity. While we have limited conscious control over its functioning, it is possible to practise forms of self-regulation which will actually moderate the ANS and in so doing enhance not only our physical functioning but also our sense of general well being (see Relaxation, pages 138–146).

Knowledge of the control system and its many different and interpenetrating levels allows us some insight into how we begin to insert a sense of 'I' into our performance. It allows us to connect with the place in us which chooses to perform. It allows us to participate more fully in learning new skills, interrupting old habits and acquiring new ones. Conscious participation in this process speeds the learning experience and enhances the sense of accomplishment at whatever level you find yourself in your sport or activity.

The key to peaceful co-existence with your control system when making strong, sustained or unusual demands upon your body, is cooperation. Cooperation with its strengths and limitations produces intelligent and efficient efforts. You use your body as it is meant to be used and you get maximum results with minimum efforts: the goal of every athlete.

Physical Goals

Strength

Muscular strength can be defined as the maximum force or tension exerted by a person in a single effort as measured by a calibrated instrument or by the single lift or resistance. Until recently, for most of us, 'strength' conjured up visions of the Amazing Hulk overturning cars and playing baseball with a telephone pole or else glistening, oiled, musclebound weightlifters parading on stage but unable to scratch their backs. Until the last decade or so most competitive athletes left weight training to the body builder for fear that such training would leave them 'musclebound', 'stiff', 'inflexible' and unable to perform the skills required by their sport.

Ample research in the 1960s dispelled these myths and demonstrated that systematic strength training regimes specific to the muscle group requirements of an individual's sport, when combined with a modest programme of flexibility training, significantly increased the speed and power of movement, and ultimately performance. The burgeoning strength training programmes on the health and fitness scene testify to the fact that the transition from the Amazing Hulk to Nautilus is now fully fledged. On the one hand there is a growing number of bodybuilders (both men and women) pursuing muscle bulk and definition through weight training, and, on the other hand, a rising tide of serious competitors who are recognizing the benefits of specific weight training in improving their performance whether it be bettering their position on the squash ladder, increasing the power of their jumps in preparation for a dance audition, or sustaining their performance on a windsurfer in a strong wind.

Having said that, continued research efforts to systematize regimes of weight training have produced more questions than answers. It is no longer clear which systems are most effective nor that results are always consistent. What is clear is that the principle of *specificity* (see Training Principles, page 146) is paramount.

Whatever the system or the motivation, strength training programmes are treading on the heels of aerobics and keep-fit classes in the popularity stakes. This being the case, there is every reason for learning how to train efficiently, effectively and safely. The guidelines laid out in 'Training Principles' are particularly relevant to strength training. However, there are several different ways of increasing the strength of a given muscle and each kind of strength reflects a different use of the body. The kind of strength you want to develop will reflect the kind of exercise you practise: isotonic, isometric, isokinetic, or variable resistance training.

Elements of strength

Strength is the maximum force which can be generated by a muscle or muscle group. It is the ability to climb stairs, lift objects, throw projectiles, etc.

Muscle bulk or hypertrophy results from regular strength training. As described in The Power System, Fast Twitch muscle fibres are more subject to increase in size through training. But the specific goal of primarily increasing muscle bulk requires a specialized training programme. High calibre bodybuilders practise more sets in a training session: from 5–10 per muscle group and include more repetitions: 8–16 in each set. This longer repetition and increased demand placed on the muscle cells results in more usage and hence an increase in their bulk. The individual who, on the other hand, wants to increase his strength (like the power lifters in the Olympics) will train with the goal of lifting heavier and heavier weights rather than lighter weights more frequently. Once again the closer your training mirrors the actual movement required, the greater the reward of the training.

Power is defined in terms of the speed at which you can produce force. In other words, a powerful person can make a strong muscular exertion very fast. Sports like the hammer throw, shotput and javelin all require substantial power. In order to increase power an individual must train in high force workouts using very heavy weights *whilst* training with as much velocity as possible. Please note, though, that it is always important in such activities that high speed training include particular emphasis on appropriate technique.

Explosive power includes an extra emphasis on speed. A slap shot in ice hockey, a goal kick in soccer, a karate punch all reflect explosive strength. In other words explosive power is strength amplified by speed. The training of Fast Twitch muscle fibres enters into the development of explosive power in movement. In addition, it is very important that explosive power be cultivated with a high degree of skill and neuro-muscular coordination. In order to have explosive power it is really necessary actually to practise the specific activity so as to coordinate the neuromuscular skill with the strength developed through strength training techniques. Once again the training principle of specificity applies.

Muscular endurance is a different quality of strength from those described here and will be discussed in the next section on endurance training.

Isotonic training

Isotonic muscular contractions are the most common of all muscular contractions. Most of our daily activities like walking, running, dressing and eating, involve isotonic movements. These take the form of either *concentric* movements where muscles actively shorten in order to overcome resistance, like curling a barbell or lifting a fork to the mouth, or *excentric*, in which the muscle is active whilst lengthening, for instance in lowering the barbell or returning the fork back to the plate. Most isotonic training will incorporate both concentric and excentric movements. In any case, the weight lifted or lowered remains constant though the speed of movement may vary. In strength training programmes the classic piece of equipment and still the most universally used is the barbell.

Two physicians, Dr Delorme and Dr Watkins, while rehabilitating injured Second World War veterans, developed a form of Progressive Resistance Exercise (PRE) which became the standard for all strength training systems and is known as the Delorme System. They developed a key concept known as the Repetition Maximum (RM). An RM is the maximum load a muscle group can lift a given number of times before fatiguing. If an individual can lift a given weight only one time before fatiguing, then that is a 1RM weight for that muscle group. If another person can lift the same weight five times before fatiguing, then that weight is a 5RM load for that person for that particular muscle group. The beauty of this form of measurement is that it is subjective. It varies according to the strength of the individual. This then enabled Delorme and Watkins to standardize a system which could be applied to all individuals. For any muscle group to be trained they worked out the following protocol:

First set of 10 repetitions: Use 50% of 10RM weight
Second set of 10 repetitions: Use 75% of 10RM weight
Third set of 10 repetitions: Use 100% of 10RM weight

So, for example, if the weight you can lift with a particular muscle group for ten repetitions before fatigue is 80lb, your 10RM would be 80lb. Following the Delorme system you would first lift a weight of 40lb (50 per cent of your RM of 80lb) ten times. This would constitute a set of ten × 50% 10RM. The next set of ten repetitions after a rest or other exercises would be 60lb (75 per cent of your 10RM of 80lb). The third set of ten repetitions would be at 80lb (100 per cent of your RM of 80lb). The way in which this system meets the overload principle of training (see page 00) is both safe and effective. When you train at a certain RM over a period of time your muscle strength increases to the point where you can lift the same weight without fatigue. You then increase the weight load to the point where you *can* only lift it ten times before fatigue. This new weight then becomes your 10RM. In this way the principle of progression is introduced into your training.

While the majority of today's isotonic training programmes follow the general principles of the Delorme system of PRE, some recommend as few as two sets of 3RMs at 100 per cent, whereas others espouse one set of 10RMs at 100 per cent. All this can be very confusing, but as an individual in training you will be able to find the best programme of PRE to suit your needs. Generally, you will be safe in your isotonic training programme if it consists of between one and three sets of repetitions and 3RM to 9RM loads.

Early on in weight training programmes, significant results accrue easily. Within the first 8–12 weeks an untrained person can expect to improve approximately 30 per cent in strength. But, in accordance with the law of diminishing returns, the more you train the more effort you have to put in to get the same rate of results. It does seem to be the case that higher intensity (heavier loads), lower repetition techniques produce greater muscle bulk than low intensity/high repetition systems which are used for endurance purposes. In any event, to get strength training results you should use at least 70 per cent of your maximum power at some point in the training programme.

Isometric training

Isometric training involves muscular contractions against a fixed, immovable load or resistance. There is no change in muscle length. Standing in a door frame and pushing against the jamb is an example of an isometric exercise. We use a variety of isometric contractions in our daily lives: straining to open the lid of a new jar of peanut butter, opening a window which has been closed all winter, pushing a stalled car up a hill. A number of sports such as water skiing, wind surfing, downhill skiing, gymnastics and wrestling all require strong isometric contractions.

A while back there was a wave of fervent isometric exercising as a result of the claims made by two German scientists, Hettinger and Müller, that strength could be increased by an average of 5 per cent a week when isometric contractions were held for as little as once a day for 6 seconds at two thirds of the maximum strength. Subsequently these claims were found to be unjustified but they sparked a surge of interest and research. It is possible to practise isometric contraction at only 50–70 per cent of maximal effort and, in fact, a number of systems definitely recommend below 100 per cent maximal contraction. But generally speaking contractions of below 50 per cent do not seem to generate substantial increases in muscular strength.

Subsequent research by Müller suggests that holding 5 to 10 near maximal contractions, for example on a bullworker exerciser, for 5–10 seconds is the most practical system. Like other training systems, isometric programmes seem to be effective when practised 3–5 days a week.

Isometric training has one great limitation. It is very specific. A muscle group trained isometrically only demonstrates its full strength when the muscle is used in a similar isometric contraction in your sport or activity and *particularly* at the joint angle at which the isometric strength was developed. If you practise isometric strengthening of your arm flexors with your elbow bent at 90 degrees, then your arm will demonstrate strength at that specific angle but there will be no substantial increase in strength at 60 or 120 degree angles of your joint. It is common in isometric training systems, therefore, to train a given muscle group with the joint at several different angles so as to 'spread the strength around'. Some training programmes for specific sports, for example waterskiing and gymnastics, will incorporate isometric exercises into an isotonic regime. This has the advantage of training muscle groups through their range of movement isotonically and then including isometric training at specific joint angles or body positions where the performer may have to sustain the contractions of a muscle group over a period of time, for example holding the rope on a run-up to the ramp at ski jumping or a held position in a gymnastics routine.

One of the advantages of isometric training is that it requires very little equipment and can be performed almost anywhere. Thus its adaptability to circumstances makes it a handy tool to take with you wherever you may be.

Isokinetic training and varying resistance training

Isokinetic training employs devices which regulate the speed of a contraction in a muscle group to a constant rate.

To achieve proper isokinetic training the *speed of contraction* must be constant so that no matter how much tension is produced in the contracting muscle the speed will be the same throughout the range of movement. With isotonic training the maximal effort is only exerted at the point where the muscle is weakest. Varying resistance or accommodation equipment, on the other hand, employs levers, hydraulic arrangements, cams and other mechanical constructions to provide varying resistance at any speed. Though similar to isokinetic equipment in their training effect they are not genuinely isokinetic. The defining characteristic of isokinetic training comes from the fact that the muscle is exercised equally, at the same percentage of its strength through the complete range of movement not just at the weakest or 'sticking' point. While there is a wide range of equipment now available with varying degrees of isokinetic 'characteristics', it is important to emphasize that the true definition of isokinetic is the *same speed* throughout the range of movement. Machines, like Nautilus, which vary the amount of *effort* required to draw the weight through your range of movement are not truly isokinetic in that you *can* vary the speed: these are in fact varying resistance machines. But the training effect such machines produce can be close enough to that of the complicated and inordinately expensive isokinetic equipment, such as Cybex, to be considered as a basic training approach instead of 'true' but rarer isokinetic training.

Whereas varying resistance training at slow speeds increases strength at slow movement speeds, varying resistance training at fast speeds increases strength at all speeds. It follows that the strength developed by performing varying resistance exercises at a fast speed will cover the wide range of movement speeds you may need to use in your exercise, sport or activity.

The general guidelines discussed for practising Progressive Resistance Exercise in the isotonic training section also apply for isokinetic and varying resistance training. Where manufacturers of equipment offer recommendations it is probably wise to follow them. However, do watch that a recommendation for a single set of repetitions is not prompted by a desire on the part of the owner of the equipment to get you on and off the equipment rapidly so as to get the highest turnover possible!

Although varying resistance and isokinetic training are ideal for strengthening muscles evenly throughout their range of movement, most of our daily activities are in fact isotonic. Consequently the training principle of specificity enters again. While some sports do require varying resistance kinds of strength, as in the case of the arm stroke in freestyle swimming, and so benefit from isokinetic or varying resistance training, most of our activities use predominantly isotonic movement patterns. So for improving physical performance in sports, dance, martial arts and other similar activities, isotonic training will provide strength most relevant to the ways in which we normally move.

A few years ago in the USA, and more recently in Britain, varying resistance training systems could do no wrong. They were the blue-eyed boys of the exercise boom: the most scientific, most effective, most equitable and coincidentally most expensive (therefore perhaps inevitably 'the best') system going. A Nautilus or Universal in everyone's gym was *de rigueur*. Currently there is a re-examination of the plusses and minuses of varying resistance training. Many exercise physiologists and sports trainers are recommending a return to isotonic training systems.

So, what should you practise – isotonic, isometric, varying resistance or isokinetic systems? The simplest guideline to follow is that of specificity. Whichever form of training mirrors the kind of activity you are pursuing will produce the most effective results. Swimmers would benefit from variable resistance training to develop strong arms for a constant stroke speed. In judo, on the other hand, which also calls for a strong upper body, your arms will need to vary their power and speed during a throw, and their strength would be improved best through isotonic training.

In summary, most Olympic athletes and professional sports people seem to prefer isotonic and free weight training. But perhaps the best recommendation is a judicious mixture of all three systems in relation to your specific sport or activity. Substantive research indicates that all three forms of training are beneficial when followed along appropriate guidelines.

Endurance

Endurance can be defined as the ability to maintain performance or work at a sustained level over a prolonged period of time. The limits of human endurance are being continually extended. Every month we hear of some new record being broken: athletes running from one end of a continent to another, cross-country skiers skiing hundreds of miles a day. The 1980 winner of the Hawaiian triathlon swam the 2.4 mile ocean leg in approximately 51 minutes, raced his bicycle around the 112 mile circumference of Oahu in 5 hours, and then ran the Hawaiian marathon leg in 3½ hours. He set a new world record for this event of 9 hours and 24 minutes. The previous record, set only the year before, was 11 hours and 15 minutes.

Running, swimming, cycling, cross-country skiing have surged to the forefront of recreational sports and for a good reason: endurance activities increase the general level of health and specifically have been proven to mitigate the risk factors of the number one killer of the post-war generations: heart disease. Under different conditions effective endurance training can improve the strength of the heart, increase blood volume and haemoglobin content in the body, reduce systolic and diastolic levels of blood pressure (see page 62), lower the resting heart rate, help control cholesterol count, control weight levels and generally contribute to a sense of well being and an enhanced quality of life.

In endurance training there are two levels at which the training effect takes place: *cardiovascular* and *muscular*.

Cardiovascular and muscular endurance training go hand in hand but different forms of exercise may selectively improve the endurance qualities of different muscle groups. In cycling, for example, the leg muscles are trained more than the arms, and in swimming there is particular emphasis on upper body endurance. Physiological changes in the actual muscle fibres of the legs versus the arms will result in their different abilities to function aerobically, but *in either case* cardiovascular training will take place.

Cardiovascular conditioning

You will remember that the mechanism for delivering energy to the body is the cardiovascular respiratory system: heart, lungs, and blood vessels. Consistent endurance training will have significant effects on the structure and functioning of this system which will in turn improve your endurance performance.

We have seen, when discussing the cardiovascular system (The Energy System, pages 58–71) how a strong heart works more efficiently at providing the muscles with oxygen-carrying blood. Because the heart size increases, blood volume increases, the left ventricle's stroke volume is increased and empties more fully with each beat and this means that the muscles are able to draw on greater oxygen supplies and therefore continue working aerobically at a higher level for longer before their anaerobic threshold is reached.

Training also increases the respiratory function of the individual. There is an increase in the VO_2Max as well as the vital capacity of the lungs. Furthermore, through training over a period of time you learn to maintain your work level during training at higher and higher percentages of your VO_2Max without pushing your energy delivery system out of aerobic energy production and back into the less efficient lactic acid system. Trained endurance runners can function at 75–80 per cent of their VO_2Max over most of a race. Some marathon runners can function at close to 90 per cent of their VO_2Max for most of the two hours of the race!

The effects of training also become very noticeable in daily life. At rest you have a slower heart rate because it takes less beats to provide all the necessary nutrients and oxygen to the body. Forty beats a minute is not uncommon among endurance athletes (as against an average of 70 beats per minute). Your training heart rate tends to decrease: you are able to get more work done with a slower heart rate. Delivery of blood (hence oxygen and energy) to the muscles is enhanced. There is an increase in the number of capillaries which means both that the diffusion distance for oxygen to get to the actual muscle fibres is shortened and also that during vasodilation (which happens whenever you begin to do exercise) there is less work on your heart. As a result blood pressure is also lowered – both systolic and diastolic blood pressure is decreased during rest and sub-maximal exercise.

In short, your heart and lungs become more efficient, stronger and better at what they are meant to do. You can achieve the same results with less effort, or better results with equal effort. The bonus is that at rest your heart and lungs have to work less hard. The risk from heart disease is substantially reduced.

Muscular endurance

There are specific physiological changes in the muscles which result from consistent, specific endurance training:

1   Muscle fibre adapts to endurance training. While the actual number of Slow Twitch and Fast Twitch muscle fibres doesn't change (see page 77), there is an increase in the proportional volume of Slow Twitch or endurance fibres in those muscles used in the endurance training. Furthermore, all fibre types, particularly the intermediate ones, develop their full aerobic potential.

2   Trained endurance muscles are more efficient at oxidizing both glucose and fat more completely. There is less resultant lactic acid build-up which will in turn mean that endurance time is prolonged and the onset of fatigue is retarded.

3   Your ability to generate ATP (the main energy supply in the muscle) aerobically is increased because the mitochondria – the powerhouses of your muscle cells – increase in number, size and efficiency (see page 77). The difference in potential for helping to generate ATP aerobically in mitochondria can be as much as four times greater in a trained endurance athlete than in an untrained individual.

4   The myoglobin (a relative of haemoglobin) in the skeletal muscle is increased by up to 80 per cent through endurance training. Consequently the quantity of available oxygen in the muscle cells at any moment is increased. The oxygen which is required to sustain aerobic activity is more consistently available and in larger quantities.

5   In endurance trained muscles the ability both to mobilize and to oxidize fat is increased. In sustained aerobic work the percentage of fat used as a source of energy becomes increasingly important as the activity is extended over a period of time. As a result of endurance training an athlete is able to maintain energy production at high levels for an entire race or competition.

If your goal is a general improvement of your overall fitness level and specifically your cardiovascular system, then any aerobic training will provide adequate conditioning as long as you follow proper guidelines.

When you train for endurance in your sport, the muscles involved automatically improve their endurance capacity as well as the cardiovascular system. However, while it is possible to enhance cardiovascular fitness through any endurance or aerobic training such as swimming, cycling, running, skipping or cross-country skiing, the training effect for muscles follows the principle of specificity. Long distance swimming may improve your cardiovascular fitness but it will not have the same direct training effect on your leg muscles as running or cross-country skiing.

If your goal is a marked improvement in your endurance sport, then your training should include not only general cardiovascular training but also specific endurance training of the muscle groups involved in the actual activity for which you are training.

Training guidelines

The amount of training one should do and the resultant amount of improvement one can expect will depend upon how fit you are to begin with. In studies of middle-aged, sedentary men with heart disease potential, maximal aerobic power improved by 50 per cent when they underwent a training programme similar to that of normal, healthy adults who only improved 10–15 per cent under the same regime. But equally, an improvement of 2–3 per cent in the aerobic capacity of an elite athlete is just as significant as an improvement of 20–30 per cent in sedentary adults.

Whatever your level of fitness, there are three variables involved in endurance conditioning which must be taken into account in order to produce effective cardiovascular and muscular conditioning.

Intensity The results you achieve from endurance training depend directly upon the intensity of the endurance overload you place upon your body. 'Overload', that is, increasing the demand upon a body function beyond what has been previously required, is a basic conditioning principle. Some of the variables which are influenced by the intensity of your endurance training include: the amount of oxygen used, since endurance training is primarily aerobic in nature; the speed at which your heart beats; the ability to minimize the use of lactic acid energy systems during performance; the onset of premature fatigue plus a host of other physiological factors. The single measurement which reflects your ability to perform optimally in endurance activities is your VO_2Max. (See page 65). Measurement of VO_2Max is a standard test for endurance capacity. The percentage of one's VO_2Max which is being utilized at any given time is directly reflected in the percentage of one's maximum heart rate. Too high a heart rate reflects workload demands which will push you beyond your anaerobic threshold. Consequently by monitoring your heart beat you are able to monitor the percentage of your VO_2Max you are using and so regulate the level of intensity at which you are training, keeping it below your anaerobic threshold.

But how fast should you work your heart? In order to achieve a training effect you have to cross a threshold which is approximately 60 per cent of your maximum heart rate. But as a safety guideline, it is best not to train at over 80 per cent of your maximum heart rate. So, it can be said that if you train at between 60 and 80 per cent of your maximum heart rate you will be training at a level of intensity which will achieve adequate cardiovascular and muscular conditioning. There is a simple formula to calculate both your maximum heart rate and establish the 60 and 80 per cent boundaries of your 'training sensitive zone':

Take the number 220 and subtract your age from it. Multiply this figure by 60 per cent and 80 per cent. As long as your heart beat stays between these two figures, you will be training within a safe but effective level of intensity. For example, if I am 30 years old, I would calculate:

$220 - 30 = 190$

$190 \times .60$ 114 (minimum level of heart beats per minute)

$190 \times .80$ 152 (maximum level of heart beats per minute)

As long as my heart beats do not fall below 114 beats per minute or rise above 152 beats per minute I will be training at a level within my Training Sensitive Zone. Pulse rates are usually taken during or immediately after training at the radial (wrist), carotid (neck) or temporal (temple) arteries. To get as accurate a result as possible you must check your pulse immediately upon stopping – even a 10-second delay can result in a marked fall in your pulse rate. The effectiveness of this simple system lies in the fact that it is a subjective measure of each individual's level of performance in relation to their own potential, not some external standard. If you are new to endurance training or unfit, a relatively low intensity training programme will still result in your heart rate creeping up towards the 80 per cent level of your maximum heart rate. As the endurance programme begins to take effect, you will have to perform more work in order to raise your heart rate to the same level. Your cardiovascular system has become more efficient. *So you will have to increase the intensity of your training in order to get the same training results.*

Consequently, maintaining your heart rate between these two thresholds will also ensure that you follow another training principle: progressiveness. You will place upon your cadiovascular system increasingly more demands all still safely within the 80 per cent threshold.

If you are unfit, it is advised to work nearer the 60 per cent threshold; if you are fit, closer to the 80 per cent threshold. It is actually very hard work for an elite athlete to train at an 80 per cent plus level because his cardiovascular system has become so efficient at what it does.

Duration How long should you train in a given session? A minimum of 20 minutes exercise at an elevated heart rate is necessary to achieve a cardiovascular conditioning. If you are a beginner and have a relatively low level of fitness, are very overweight or have a heart condition, then this is a good level to start at. However, as soon as it is comfortable, moving on to 30 minute sessions will provide a training effect which will be more enduring and enhance your fitness level more effectively. For the fit individual, duration can be extended to 40–100 minutes of uninterrupted exercise. If you train at higher levels of intensity, say 75–85 per cent of maximum heart rate, then a sustained session of 30–60 minutes should result in substantial endurance conditioning. Remember 100 minutes of uninterrupted training activity is a lot. A pre-marathon run of 12–16 miles would still fall within this 100 minute limit!

Frequency There is constant debate about how often one should train. Opinions vary from as few as two to as many as seven days a week. Some studies on interval training show that two days a week of training produced the same changes in the VO₂Max level as those observed in a 5-day a week training schedule. In other studies there was no significant difference in the training results when individuals trained for two versus four days, or in other studies, three versus five days, *as long as the total work accomplished was held constant*. 'Hidden exercise', like walking up stairs, shopping, etc, are all proving relevant as well.

Generally speaking, most people agree that, as a basic guideline, endurance training at an adequate level of intensity can be achieved over three to five days a week for 30 minutes a session. This will result in consistent improvement in VO₂Max and is often recommended as a basic training routine for an average individual seeking an improved level of fitness. Top athletes train six or seven days a week and may run up to 20 miles a day, breaking it up into two sessions: perhaps an 8 mile run in the morning and a 12 mile run in the afternoon. A long distance runner at the peak of his training period might run anywhere from 120 to 160 miles a week.

Intensity, duration and frequency must all be considered when you organize your training regime. Each factor can be manipulated as long as: intensity is at least 60 per cent of your maximum heart rate; duration is at least 20 minutes in a training session; and frequency is at least twice a week. In order to continue to enhance your cardiovascular fitness you must bear in mind the principles of *progressive training* and *maintenance of an overload*. This can be achieved by manipulating the three training factors so that you sustain an overload on your cardiovascular system to which you continue to adapt and therefore progressively increase. Strict endurance training can be boring so play with the three control factors in order to enliven your training.

Training approaches

Interval training has been the most common form of athletic training throughout the years. It consists of repetitions of a given training distance or speed several times with rest intervals between each distance. A runner might run 220 yards four times, then 440 yards four times, then 110 yards twice. There are several variables which can be adjusted in interval training:

Work interval: the portion of the interval training programme during which you actually work.

Rest interval: the time between work intervals.

Set: this is a group of work and rest intervals. An example would be four 220 runs, each at 30 seconds with four 45-second rest intervals.

Repetitions: this is the number of times you work in a set. In the above example, there are four repetitions in a set.

Training time: in order to get maximal benefit out of interval training it is important that the work/rest interval times be maintained. Of course as you near the end of a set or training session, it is more difficult to maintain the same speed for a work interval or not slip into longer rest intervals.

Trainers talk about an 'interval prescription'. This is a formula of several different interval sets designed to meet your individual needs and the training requirements of your particular sport or event. Because there are so many variables which can be manipulated, it is easy, with knowledgeable coaching, to prescribe the right combination of factors for each individual which can be adjusted as your fitness level increases during a season. Whichever endurance sport you engage in, proper prescriptions of interval sessions can be developed for you. While interval training has traditionally been used more for sprinters it has definite benefits for endurance activities as well. Swimming, cycling and soccer all use interval training. In the martial arts, interval training could be said to take the form of katas: prescribed, formalized training routines.

Fartlek This form of endurance training was developed by the Swedish coach, Gosta Holmer, in the 1930s. Roughly translated it means 'speed play'. One of the real problems with interval training (which anyone who participated in school athletics will surely remember) is the inevitable and sometimes oppressive boredom which accompanies the day after day cranking out of the inexorable sets. In Fartlek training, there is no prescribed interval. Fast sprints may be interspersed with slower distance. Work intervals vary in length. Often rest intervals are taken as slow jogs, or in the case of cycling gentle pedalling over flat terrain.

The main benefits of Fartlek training is that the athlete works according to how he or she feels at the time. This creates a genuine sense of freedom and spontaneity as well as flexibility in the training routine. Early season injuries are usually minimal. It is particularly adaptable to the serious but essentially non-competitive goals of many people. It is also particularly suitable for outdoor training, for runners, skiers, cyclists, etc, where the rhythm and pace of the training can be varied as the landscape changes.

There are two main disadvantages. It is difficult to monitor training benefits 'scientifically', there being no rigorous way of measuring results or setting goals. Secondly, there is no external source of motivation like time objectives, limited rest intervals, assigned repetitions, etc. It is left up to self-motivation to determine how it 'feels' and whether or not you can increase the demands made upon yourself in order to satisfy the overload principle in your training. None the less, it offers good opportunities for varying the pace and speed of training. For serious competitors it is a favourite form of 'off season' training in which you can keep in shape, continue to train and yet 'play' with your training at the same time.

Long slow distance (LSD) training   This form of endurance training, which is used most often by long distance and marathon runners, was first clearly formulated by Dr Ernst van Aaken. He called it a 'pure endurance method'. Joe Henderson in *Runners World* first coined the term 'LSD' running when he made a case for running not having to be painful in order to produce results. Harols Norpoth, former European and World Record holder of the five kilometre run uses this system as do many of the contemporary leaders in the marathon world like Alberto Salazar.

In LSD training the distance must be long and relatively uninterrupted by rest intervals. The intensity of the work must be maintained within your training sensitive zone (i.e. maintaining a pulse rate of between 60 and 80 per cent of your maximum heart rate). As training proceeds you should move your training near to the 80 per cent threshold and the distance of the course should approach the length of the competition. 'Mile' runners might run several miles at a consistent rate whereas marathon runners might train at about half the distance of a marathon each day. While it has been used mostly by runners, the advantages of this system for other long-distance sports like cycling, rowing and cross-country skiing are obvious. LSD training is a valuable way for beginners to train. Individuals at risk of coronary heart disease should practise this system rather than interval or circuit training. It is also a break from the rigours of a tough interval training schedule, a good off-season form of training for middle distance runners and a relatively easy way to begin pre-season training.

Circuit training   This form of training (described in detail in Body Conditioning Methods (see pages 187–212) is often used as a part of endurance training because of its great flexibility and adaptability. It helps break up the monotonous interval training regime with circuits which work on strengthening specific muscle groups, weight training techniques which focus on strengthening the endurance muscles, or stations placed around the perimeter of a field which consist of various gymnastic or free form exercises (such as press ups). Alternatively a circuit training regime, as a change of pace from running or swimming, can be practised one or two days a week focusing on improving endurance of those muscle groups involved in the sport.

Most research suggests that all four systems of training when practised regularly, conscientiously, and with an eye to maintaining proper frequency, duration and intensity, seem to produce the results desired by the athlete. There is no conclusive evidence that one system has a distinct advantage over another if the athlete is motivated and trains appropriately. Certainly, when considering a training regime we would suggest that you follow a system to begin with which most suits your mentality, lifestyle and means. A judicious mixture of all systems works well and as one system grows stale or inadequate, another can be used to replace or relieve it temporarily or over the long term.

Flexibility

Everyone agrees that suppleness is an essential component of physical well being and that a free, full range of movement will enhance physical performance in almost all activities, from dance and gymnastics through running, tennis and skiing to karate and tae kwon do. In some cases, like ballet or gymnastics, flexibility is essential. It goes without saying that it formed a cornerstone of Nureyev's dance technique or Olga Korbut's milestone Olympic performance. For most sports and activities it is a valuable addition to training regimes. For holistic systems like yoga, it forms the core of the physical aspect of the training.

Most runners, be they the 30 minute no-more-no-less fat fighter, the regular cardiovascular fitness enthusiast, or the serious marathoner, make a show of some kind of stretching before they begin their run. For some it may be no more than a swivel of the hips and a few token bobs of head and hands towards the toes. For the serious it may involve fifteen or twenty minutes of limbering up and a decent stretching routine. But everyone agrees: stretching is good for you. If nothing else it will help prevent stiffness after training.

Flexibility is one of those things which you notice when you don't have it. Whether bending down to pick up an object, struggling with your forward bend in yoga or pulling a muscle when you reach low for a tennis backhand, flexibility is conspicuous in its absence. When working through the aftermath of an injury we are aware of how stiff we have become, how much ground we have lost in our level of flexibility. In all of these cases we quickly come to realise that flexibility is an essential element of optimal physical performance and general well being.

Flexibility is increased by stretching. But there is stretching and there is stretching. Simply adding stretching exercises to a training regime may not always be valuable. Stretching has to be directed to the particular needs of your body and the physical goals of your sport, dance, martial art or exercise form. There is also considerable disagreement in the world of sports training and rehabilitation as to whether or not joints *should* be stretched beyond their normal range of movement as is the case in some forms of hatha yoga and many dance systems. It is possible that injuries occur as much through hypermobility (extreme flexibility) as through rigidity or restricted range of movement. And as often as not injuries are caused by the actual stretching itself. Dr Richard Domingues, a well-known American orthopaedic surgeon and sports physician says: 'I hear people blaming running for back problems when they should be blaming the stretching they do before starting out. Stretching is a significant cause of injuries.' Indeed. But Domingues' indictment applies to stretching done incorrectly, in particular static stretching. But we believe that a long, slow stretch performed correctly, at the right time, can significantly enhance physical performance – sports or otherwise.

Stretching also improves blood circulation. As a muscle is contracted and released blood flow is encouraged, there is a more efficient elimination of toxins and waste products from the muscle cells and an increased supply of fresh oxygen to the working limb. *Stretching must be done correctly*: the right exercises, done in the right way, with the right amount of effort, at the right time in a training routine. (No, it's not as simple as a few unconscious bobs at the toes.)

Two particular aspects of the muscle are involved in stretching: the myotactic reflexes and connective tissue resistance.

Myotactic reflexes

Myotactic reflexes are part of the way your nervous system protects you from injuring your muscles. Most reflexes act as unconscious protectors of the body or coordinators of movement. They act without your having to organize the commands from higher levels of consciousness in your nervous system. If you had to think 'How?' when someone shouted at you to jump out of the way of an oncoming bus it would be too late. If you had to evaluate the sensation of pain from the burning stove and come to the conclusion that it was damaging your fingertips before withdrawing your hand you would end up with second degree burns. Furthermore, if you had to think how to keep your centre of gravity over your feet you would never be able to climb stairs or tie your shoes, never mind pirouette or traverse a ski slope. There are even dozens of reflexes in operation all the time just to keep your head straight on top of your neck.

There are two particular myotactic reflexes which are built into your muscles in order to protect them from injury when they are being stretched or worked hard: the *Stretch Reflex* and the *Golgi Tendon Organs*.

The stretch reflex is the product of 'muscle spindles' which are specialized muscle fibres within the muscle. The main function of muscle spindles is to help coordinate the movement of the muscle so it is smooth and efficient by giving constant feedback about how contracted they are and how hard they are working. This takes place during all movements, not just stretching. When a muscle is being stretched too fast or too much the muscle spindle relays information by an automatic reflex back to the spinal cord which immediately returns a signal to the muscle to contract in order to counteract the excessive stretch. The amount of contraction is directly related to the amount of stretch. The harder you stretch the more your stretch reflexes tell your muscle to contract: stalemate. Attempts to override this protective reflex lead first to warning pain signals and, if ignored, eventually injury. In order to circumvent the stretch reflex you need to move *slowly* and *gently* into the stretch position. The less you excite the involuntary contraction of the muscle the less you will have to fight against it and the more easily it will stretch.

The Golgi tendon organs are nerve receptors in the tendons which connect the muscles to the bones. They produce something called 'the inverse stretch response' which, at first sight, would seem to do the opposite of the muscle spindle. When too much pressure is exerted on the tendon by a muscle working very hard, the Golgi tendon organ brings about a reflex inhibition of the motor nerve stimulating the muscle: the muscle relaxes or lets go further in order to avoid injury to itself or its connective tissue. If you are waterskiing and fall, you reflexively let go of the handle of the rope rather than be dragged through the water and risk dislocating a shoulder.

The implications for stretching are significant. When you reach the maximum point of a stretch (not to the point of pain!), if you maintain that stretch the Golgi tendon organs will intervene and send messages to the resisting muscle to stop contracting. If you calibrate the stretch correctly this will result in a 'letting go' of the muscles which are unconsciously holding on

and resisting further stretching. Most people who have practised regular systems of stretching have experienced that point
during each of their stretches where their tension dissipates:
they 'relax' into their stretch and the muscle can then be
lengthened even a little further. This gentle extension of the
stretch which excites the Golgi tendon organs has to be coordinated with the stretch reflex of the muscle spindles so that
you don't stimulate them to pull the muscle back. It's a delicate
balancing act between two counterbalanced reflexes.

It takes a minimum of 7 seconds for this first release in a held
stretch position to happen. Recommended lengths of time for a
stretch vary from 10 seconds to 60 seconds. Yoga asanas are
often held for considerably longer. But however long you
stretch, approach it slowly, hold it gently and then *allow yourself*
to stretch a little further.

Connective tissue resistance

Muscle fibres themselves do not actually stretch a great deal.
They either contract, relax or lengthen to their full extent. It is
the connective tissue (sometimes referred to as the myofacia)
which wraps up each of the progressive strands of muscle tissue
– sacromere, muscle fibre, muscle bundle and finally the muscle
itself – that can be gently stretched. Physiologically speaking
there are two different kinds of stretch possible in connective
tissue.

Elastic stretching is characterized by a spring-like behaviour in
which the elongation of the connective tissue is recovered after
the load is reduced or work completed. The tissue springs back
to its original shape like an elastic band. It is a temporary,
recoverable elongation.

Plastic stretching is characterized by a more putty-like behaviour. The 'linear deformation' or lengthening which results
from the tensile stress (the stretch) remains after the stress is
removed. It's like stretching a piece of chewing gum. After you
stop pulling it still remains lengthened.

It should be clear that when practising a stretching routine, if
we can create conditions which allow the connective tissue to
respond in a plastic, malleable way, our stretching exercise will
be more effective and the results more enduring.

These are the factors which contribute to plastic stretching:

1   Use gentle effort and a low force stretch position. When you subject connective tissue to low force stretching it acts more like a plastic substance: it stays stretched. When you subject connective tissue to high force stretching it acts more like an elastic substance: it bounces back.
2   Warm up beforehand to raise body temperature. Under elevated temperatures your connective tissue stretches more easily and stays stretched. Under normal or colder temperatures the muscle and connective tissue bounce back to their original starting position.
3   Move slowly into your stretch position. Connective tissue acts in a more plastic way when it is subject to slow change. Slow speeds don't excite the myotactic reflexes which cause connective tissue to act in a more elastic fashion.
4   Hold your stretches. Connective tissue retains its plastic properties when held at its near maximum extension. Too rapid return to original positions results in an elastic recovery of original length.

There is another crucial consideration for your stretching routine which involves the above principles. When connective tissue is subject to high force and short duration stretching, *structural damage* takes place. But when subject to low force and slow speed stretching, structural weakening is minimal. In addition, stretching done at colder temperatures causes more structural damage than stretching done when you are warm. This is the reason why physical educators increasingly are insisting that an athlete warms up first, *before* stretching! Many coaches will suggest that an athlete stretch after a training session rather than before: the results are better and the chance of injury is less.

Approaches to stretching

There are five basic approaches to stretching, each with its own merits and shortcomings. In our opinion the first three are either less effective or require careful supervision and are open to injuries. We list them here because they are all ways of stretching commonly encountered and all of them will increase your flexibility to some degree.

Ballistic movement involves the building up of momentum through a swinging movement which uses the weight of your body to increase the force of the stretch. It is a pre-programmed movement which once initiated has no feedback control over it. Bouncing to touch your toes, windmill sweeps of the hand to the opposite toe, sitting on the floor and bouncing your chest towards your thighs to stretch your lower back are all ballistic. *It is one of the least effective forms of stretching and one of the quickest paths to injury.* Ballistic stretching creates a high, fast force, putting more than double the normal tension on the muscle. It evokes a strong stretch reflex contraction, pulling the muscle back, so shortening it; there is no time for the 'inverse stretch response' to be activated by the Golgi Tendon Organs, allowing the muscle to lengthen, and it creates an elastic response in the connective tissue causing it to spring back to its original shape. Ballistic stretches are most likely to cause structural weakness and eventually injury to the muscle, tendon, ligament, and ultimately the joint. Although common practice in keep fit and other sports, we heartily recommend that you do not use ballistic stretching. Remember that a ballet dancer who can perform endless *grand battements* can do so because she has spent long sessions of gentle, firm stretching for many years.

Passive stretching is slightly misleading as a name. It involves working with a partner who adds additional pressure or tension to your stretch. You are being stretched by the other person. *When correctly done*, it is a very strong and effective technique. Guidelines are: work carefully with a partner of roughly the same strength and size. Listen very carefully to your body in order to know when to say stop, *emphatically*. And lastly, you should practise this exercise under supervision. This form of stretching is of particular value in those sports and activities which require extreme ranges of motion like gymnastics and ballet. Yoga teachers frequently assist students in their stretching, again because of the high flexibility sought by this discipline. But in most activities, the extreme range of motion which passive stretching can foster is not required and the possible risks outweigh most of the benefits.

Contract/relax techniques actually contract the muscle to be stretched for 5–10 seconds before stretching. The reasoning behind this is that the Golgi Tendon Organs are then stimulated to fire first and entice the muscle to relax more in conjunction with the actual stretch. It sounds like a good idea. Unfortunately it is not so clear that the muscle relaxes completely after the contraction. As a result you have to overcome the residue of contraction in your stretch. A number of physicians and physio-therapists believe this kind of stretching leaves the muscle open to injury and warn against it. Interestingly, this approach is mirrored in strength training where it is called Proprioceptive Neuromuscular Technique. You stretch first, triggering the Stretch Reflex and thus making your actual muscle contraction stronger. Again the evidence is not totally convincing. Be careful of these kinds of 'booster' techniques.

In **static stretching** you move gently and slowly into the stretch position and then hold it for 30–60 seconds. It is practised by the individual with no external force or assistance. The tension exerted is only that of the muscles themselves with some help from gravity in certain positions. Of all the systems discussed so far, this is the safest. It is also effective. The reaction of the Stretch Reflex is minimalized, the length of time in the stretch is enough to allow the Golgi Tendon Organs to relax the muscle a bit more. It is a low force, long duration stretch: the kind that allows the connective tissue to assume its plastic properties and therefore stretch more and retain the stretch afterwards. Less structural weakening results in fewer cases of injury.

Dynamic range of movement may or may not be considered stretching. We think it should. In speaking out against the above forms of stretching, Dr Richard Domingues advocates range of movement exercises that are active and controlled. 'Why should you move a joint further than you can actually control it?' he asks in his belief that over-stretching muscles and ligaments around the joint sets the individual up for injury. The proposition behind range of movement stretching exercises is that the stretch is not performed in isolation but incorporated into strengthening, postural and neuromuscular training so that the flexibility achieved is within the normal usage and demands placed upon the body. This is eminently sensible for those who simply wish to enhance their suppleness and ability to lead an active life without cricking their neck if they turn quickly or feeling stiff when they rise from a chair. There is always a danger in any training programme which over-emphasizes any one of the six physical goals outlined in this chapter to the exclusion of the others. Imbalance and distortion lead to dysfunction and injury. Whatever training programme you choose to pursue it must be life enhancing before all else.

While it is questionable that there is any great benefit to be gained from *hyper*flexibility, it is clear that increased flexibility

---

Guidelines for stretching

1   Do not stretch cold. Precede a stretch with a warm-up (for example, a gentle few minutes jogging or limbering up). If it is cold, outdoors or in the studio, keep warm during the stretching with extra layers of clothing. (One of the best times to do a daily stretch is soon after getting out of bed in the morning – like cats and dogs! – as your body is warm and relaxed. It's a good way to start the day.)

2   Move into the stretch position slowly and gently. Do not hold to the point of pain.

3   Gentle force. More power is not necessarily better.

4   At the maximum point of the stretch hold for a minimum of 30 seconds.

5   Aim for proper alignment so choose stable stretch positions.

6   As part of a general workout, keep fit class or training, leave deep stretching until the middle or end (when the body is warm). You can precede the training with a gentle limbering up (e.g. gentle jogging on the spot etc.).

7   Start with gentle stretches and proceed to harder ones.

8   Alternate muscle groups. If you want to concentrate on a particular area come back to it several times during the routine with a progression of different exercises. Don't attack it!

9   Static stretching is the safest and produces good results, but explore dynamic range of movement systems which offer a more integrated approach to flexibility, such as Feldenkrais, Alexander, Mensendieck, Pilates.

and suppleness are principal contributors to well being. In addition, they guard against injury in the power sports and martial arts, thereby adding another element to superior performance. (Even boxers are known to take ballet classes!)

Neuromuscular Control

We all know someone whom we consider to be a 'natural athlete', someone who, no matter what they put their hand to, seems to accomplish it with inordinate skill, ease and proficiency. It may have seemed effortless, but the control that this person manifested was the result of a large number of variables and factors which include not only hereditary gifts but early childhood training and subsequent practice of skills. The sum total of inherent and learned capacities could be labelled 'neuromuscular control'.

Reflexes   Reflexive movements are basic compositional movements which are not generally under control of the central nervous system. As such, they are always in operation influencing and mitigating any of the learned or voluntary movements which go into any kind of physical skills. Reflex arcs were discussed in the section on the control system. The myotactic reflexes in the section on flexibility (pages 111–119) and the Righting reflexes which influence posture (pages 128) are examples of such reflexes moderating function.

Abilities   Abilities are the next level of sophistication in neuromuscular control. By and large they are genetically determined. But research and experimentation have made clear that the environment in the early period of development and the kinds of motor-learning opportunities experienced during that period influence the ability levels of a child (as well as its general level of intelligence, emotional tenor and physical health as an adult and the overall sense of 'self' and self-regulation).

There are over a hundred different abilities recognized by physical educators. When NASA carried out a battery of tests on its astronauts in which 18 primary abilities were measured, they established four major categories: 1 – fine manipulative abilities; 2 – gross positioning and movement abilities; 3 – system equalization abilities (dealing with velocity and acceleration in relation to the environment and to objects); 4 – perceptual-cognitive abilities (for example, reaction time and dividing attention between several simultaneous tasks). No individual has a corner on all the various abilities and as often as not the natural athlete excels at a sport because her particular mix of abilities suit the demands of the sport *and* because she chooses to perform those events she can do naturally.

Skills If we say that someone has innate ability, we can also describe a person as skilful in the performance of their sport or activity. A downhill skier skilfully progresses down a steep slope, a ballet dancer skilfully executes a difficult *pas de deux*, a martial artist skilfully throws an opponent. Skill might be defined as the learned ability to achieve consistently a set target with the minimum expenditure of time and energy. One of the characteristics of a skilled person is the ability to perform apparently complex activities with grace, effortlessness and smooth timing, i.e. as if it were simple. In learning a skill, we spend a protracted period of time progressing along a continuum from unskilled to skilled behaviour. Usually, then, you can say that a skill is learned whereas an ability is innate.

While a simplification, it could be said that most movement patterns consist of reflexive movements, abilities and skills.

One of the challenges of any parent or teacher is to help a child find a particular sport or activity which matches with the child's innate abilities so that he experiences success in his attempts to learn the skills which go with that sport. Everyone has certain innate abilities and if we experience early failure in sport because we are compelled to train in a sport to which we are not suited, the trauma of failure often extends to all sports or physical activities. We then develop a skill deficit in general as we avoid physical training and begin to think of ourselves as 'clumsy' or 'awkward'. Often it is simply a case that we should be playing table tennis instead of rugby football, or running instead of training in ballet.

Motor learning

Motor learning is the process whereby we train physically to use our innate abilities in order to develop skill in a particular activity. All activities will require motor learning in order to perform them. Some like downhill skiing or kung fu may require a lot of learning whereas running or keep fit classes will require much less. Through successive rehearsals of a skill you acquire more and more control over the movements required to perform it. How the control system organizes movement in the body is explained on pages 81–92. Here is how the three stages in motor learning – cognitive, associative and automatic – would apply to learning the backhand in tennis.

1 Cognitive phase   At the beginning of learning a skill you start to develop a sense of what the skill should feel like. You are learning what is actually required of you and developing some feel of how the skill goes together: in a tennis backhand you learn how to grip the racquet, where your feet should be positioned, how to begin to track the ball as it crosses the net, etc. At this point it is important to have clear and accurate information, good teaching, reading or video input, anything which helps trace the pathways in the motor cortex as clearly as possible. Individuals with a large number of innate abilities specific to a sport are often characterized by a rapid acquisition of basic skills: they learn fast.

2 Associative phase   In this phase, you now have a grasp of the basic skills required. You know where to place your feet, what angle your body should be to the net, how to follow through on your backhand. You now begin to refine the skill and move it closer towards accepted standards of correctness. By this phase, much of the learned motor behaviour is being stored in the pre-motor cortex. There is a shuttling back and forth of activity between your motor cortex where experimentation and differentiation goes on and your premotor cortex where the skill is being stored and is available for use as a whole. This is accompanied of course by intense activity in other areas of the Central Nervous System like the spine and cerebellum which are also active during movement. More of the skill has been retained and basic engrams or patterns are already laid down in your control system, so you now learn faster and the learning process is less frustrating because the skill is now actually available to you. You now not only hit the ball back over the net but you begin to direct it, controlling speed and direction.

3 Automatic phase   At this stage, you no longer have to think and consider what you are doing. The performance is automatic, the skill is fully acquired and incorporated into the performance of the sport. As a tennis player you have learned not only the backhand shot but can include either top spin or a slice into the shot. You can drive the ball to the back of your opponent's court or nudge a drop shot over the net. The backhand can be taken on the run and the placement of the ball covers the entire court.

The mind

There are certain functions which characterize the mind and which are involved in any motor learning process. While they have a physiological and biological basis, they are best understood in terms of their functions.

Attention   During physical activity we are taking in thousands of bits of information each second, yet we can focus on only a few at any given moment. The individual must select from this wide range of information those bits of it which are appropriate for the activity at hand. It is no good looking at the floor when facing your partner in an aikido drill or your opponent's hands when he attempts to dribble around you in soccer. In all activities you must find a proper balance between what you focus on and how you fit that information into the broader picture. This process is called 'filtering'. You orient and focus your attention properly so that the information you actually process is appropriate for the behaviour in which you are engaged. The cultivation of this mental ability is what we generally call good concentration. Concentration usually involves two things: the ability to sustain your attention over an extended period of time on whatever the information and neuromuscular control which will achieve the desired results; and the ability to shift your attention from internal to external and from broad to narrow focus. All things being equal in terms of skill and ability, the individual with more effective concentration will almost always outperform the individual whose concentration is sporadic.

Anticipation If attention means selecting information and then focusing on the right internal response, anticipation involves guessing what is going to happen next before it happens and initiating the right response earlier, thereby reducing the amount of reaction time required. The extra fraction of a second gained in the correct anticipation of the gun as you launch off the blocks in a sprint can make the difference in the result of the race. Knowing where your karate opponent will attack next allows you to initiate the block and the counter attack as well. Anticipating which side of the tennis court your opponent will cover results in a passing shot that leaves your opponent flat footed. There are four mental factors which constitute good anticipation: 1 – the amount of time you can anticipate, for example how long you can plan before you encounter the mogul ahead of you in your downhill ski run; 2 – spatial orientation, for example knowing where your team mates are at the other end of the soccer pitch so that your pass lands in the space towards which they are moving in a break for the goal; 3 – receptor anticipation, for example knowing when and where the ball is going to arrive to meet the face of your racquet; and 4 – effector anticipation, such as knowing how to organize your racquet swing so that the face of the racquet meets the ball on the sweet spot. These last two, receptor and effector anticipations, are the components of what is generally called 'good timing'.

Arousal There is a commonly accepted relationship between the level of arousal and performance. As arousal increases, performance increases up to a certain optimal point at which point you begin to become over-aroused and the level of performance deteriorates. This relationship is known as the *inverted U curve*, the peak of which is the level of optimal performance for the individual. Extroverts can take much more arousal and excitation than introverts, their performance is boosted by high arousal stimulation, excitement or the 'big match' situation whereas introverts are more easily aroused and too much excitation sends them over the top so that the level of their performance plummets.

In addition, the more experience you have the more you are able to deal with arousal and ride with it. If you are in-

(a) The Influence of Arousal on Performance Level

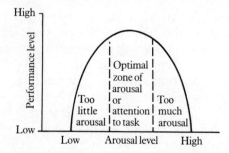

The Yerkes-Dodson Law. If arousal is very low or very high, performance will suffer. If arousal is optimum, then performance will also be at the peak.

(b) The Influence of Arousal on Beginners vs Experts

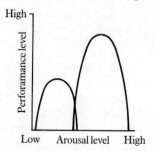

Beginners reach their peak much more quickly when arousal increases, whereas experts require more arousal and can maintain performance during high arousal states.

(c) The Influence of Arousal on Introverts vs Extroverts

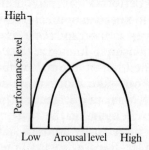

The performance of introverts suffers from high arousal whereas extroverts can maintain performance during high arousal states.

experienced, too much arousal leads to a quick drop in the level of performance. Different activities also require, and lead to, different levels of arousal. A football match will generate considerable arousal, whereas a t'ai-chi ch'uan class will require a sustained but lower level of arousal. Yoga or Feldenkrais classes are best practised with minimal arousal. Remember also that the more excited or aroused you are, the more you will need to rely upon already learned habits and acquired skills. You cannot unlearn a bad habit or acquire a new skill if you are too excited. This is because the stronger the arousal the more your Reticular Activating System will stimulate the learned and stored skills you have already acquired. Too much excitation makes it very difficult for your motor cortex to explore, differentiate and analyse movement. In addition, your sympathetic nervous system will be adding to the general level of excitation making it even more difficult to interfere or inhibit your habitual or reflexive responses. Learning must take place in a calm, supportive and not-threatening environment.

Exactly where the optimal arousal lies for an individual depends upon all of the above factors and will vary from day to day, sport to sport and individual to individual. Find your own optimal level of arousal and if necessary when over aroused use relaxation or awareness techniques to bring yourself down to that level.

Habituation We all develop habits. They are the control system's mechanism for dealing with the multitude of unconscious movement decisions we need to make throughout the day. We don't always have the luxury of reflecting on each physical activity since other subjective factors often take our full attention. In most cases the organization of our movement operates from places so deep in the unconscious mind that we are no longer even aware that we are making a movement: we may blow on our fingers before taking a tennis serve, receive and control a soccer ball with our left foot or automatically stand with our feet together in a yoga asana, without even knowing we do it.

Habits are a part of our way of delegating responsibility to other centres in the brain. By the time we have reached physical maturity, the vast majority of our movement patterns are unconscious habits. And quite rightly, as we would never be able to take the time to relearn the vast repertoire of movement patterns which constitute our daily functioning each time we needed to sit, walk, or perform a skill. The problem is that bad habits, like good habits, become familiar. So much so that when we attempt to change them, they feel 'wrong'. In order to change bad habits and replace them with correct movement we have to be aware not only of how to change a habit but what we are actually doing as well: we need feedback.

Feedback (knowledge of results)

Earlier on we discussed the three stages of motor learning: cognitive, associative and automatic. Developing effective neuromuscular control involves shifting back and forth between these three stages. But in order to improve a skill you have to have feedback on how you are doing. For example you will need feedback about your attention and concentration: noticing when you are focusing on appropriate body movements as opposed to external stimuli, for example. Or you will need to know if your sense of timing is accurate, how well you are anticipating your opponent's next move or a change in the terrain over which you are running, skiing or cycling. But in addition to this you will need feedback about three key elements of the motor skills you are practising: sequence, phasing and force.

Sequence is the order in which a movement progresses. The progression of movement in a dance jump, karate kata or a swimming stroke will always be the same. **Phasing** is the relative length of time each of the components of a complex skill takes. In golf this would break down into how long it takes to complete your backswing, how long you hold the club at the top of its arc, how fast the swing progresses, and how long you keep your head down as you follow through. Of course as you shift from a fairway wood to a gentle chip or a putt, the phasing of the movement will change. **Force** is the third element. You can vary the force in the different components of a skill and this will influence the end result. A slice and a drop shot in tennis are similar, but by exerting different force in each shot, the end result is competely different. In running more than anywhere else it is possible to see how important the influence of sequence, phasing and force is. Walking, jogging, running a six-minute mile, running a four-minute mile, running the 400 metres or sprinting the 100 metres all use the same basic skill only it is adapted, changed and modified as the speed and pace change according to the situation and the length of the race.

There are at least six factors which influence your knowledge of results, or feedback. **Kinaesthetic information** is essential. You need to *feel* what you are doing and how your body is performing. Time spent in awareness techniques and general sensitization will help improve your ability to get the most information from your practice of skills.

As you become more familiar with your skills and techniques, you should be able to rely more substantially on **internal self-regulation** over external information. You learn how to listen to your body.

Input from the outside, from your coach or colleagues, for example, should be as accurate as possible. General comments like: 'good', or 'that's right', provide little useful feedback as to what is 'good' or what is 'right'. Look for specific and accurate feedback: 'Your follow-through is good', 'your spine is not straight in that yoga asana', etc.

After feedback is given, there must be **time to practise** it and explore what that means in physical terms, before giving more information. Feedback overload is confusing and can be more harmful than too little feedback. Digest input before taking in more.

Allow for **regular rest or relaxation intervals** during an extended training. Too lengthy training sessions result in tiredness, loss of concentration, and decreasing ability to retain new skills as they are experienced. You can actually ruin a valuable training session by not stopping when tired but continuing on and consequently practising sloppy, incorrect technique.

Practice with accurate feedback and detailed knowledge of results will lead to increased control over skills and a general improvement in performance. **Proper practice and proper feedback produce proper results.**

Posture

Posture is a word we all use to descibe some elusive body state. For most of us it seems to have something to do with standing straight, chest out, buttocks tucked under, shoulders back and all the other misguided notions of posture which have sprung out of our military traditions. The ideas of early gymnastic teachers like Jahn and Ling and the German and Scandinavian military training traditions are still prejudicing our thoughts about posture long after we have abandoned their jumping jacks and windmill toe-touching routines which cause so much damage and do so little good.

The main problem with teaching posture is that it is thought of as a position, something static. The Latin words *ponere* and *positura* refer to a static position and foster the misconception of holding a rigid alignment in the body. So before trying to discuss the body mechanics of posture let's redefine it. Moshe Feldenkrais, one of the pioneers of movement re-education methods has this to say:

> One can assume a good position while having a bad posture because posture is concerned with the way the good or bad position is achieved. . . . Posture describes the use of the entire self in achieving and maintaining this or that change of configuration and position . . . the way the effect, the motivation, the direction, and the execution of the act is organized while it is being performed. (*Potent Self*)

The key to good posture then is not only correct alignment, but the way that the alignment is achieved and maintained whatever position one is in.

The body as an anti-gravity mechanism

All movement takes place in gravity and with our unique upright posture we are more susceptible to the influence of gravity than any other animal. Our skeleton can be seen as a system of levers, and our muscles are the source of power which move the skeleton and help keep it erect. We are constantly maintaining this erect position in spite of gravity. So our body can be seen as an anti-gravity mechanism.

Fortunately over 90 per cent of the control of movement in

humans is unconscious and a large part of the organization of our balance and equilibrium in a standing position takes place in these unconscious parts of the brain. This is even more the case with our anti-gravity mechanisms which is just as well since we couldn't possibly orchestrate all the minutiae of movement, coordination and balance consciously.

These self-regulating mechanisms would maintain a balanced upright posture if they were not interfered with by bad habits learned as we grow up. These shorten or collapse the body in a way which makes the anti-gravity battle a losing one. For our body's reflexive and natural anti-gravity functions to assert themselves, we need to interrupt bad habits: like hunching the shoulders which causes restricted range of movement in the neck and a congested shoulder girdle; or collapsing the upper chest which inhibits proper breathing; or standing with a sway back which causes lower back pain and restricts the movement of the diaphragm and the easy assimilation of food in the intestines; or restricting movement in the pelvis and hips which limits general mobility and can cause sexual dysfunction. Equally important, we would then not have to compensate by trying to 'stand tall', or 'straighten our back', or 'tuck in our pelvis', which only overlays and restricts the proper anti-gravity functions and brings more inner conflict. It would seem, in true Zen fashion, that 'not doing' is the best way to sustain correct posture: less effort, less resistance, less inner conflict.

The body: a balancing act

The body's upright posture is achieved by piling up the different parts of the body one on top of the other: The head and neck on the torso, the torso and spine on the pelvis, and the pelvis on the legs and feet. In a way the body is stacked up like three pyramids, with the apex of each pyramid balancing on the base of the one below it.

The pelvis – the base for movement
The pelvis is both the base upon which the upper body is supported and at the same time the main source of power for locomotion. It provides stability so that the upper body can function with ease and disregard for what is happening below,

while maintaining power and mobility in its own movement. It is symmetrical and each side is made up of three fused bones: the pubis, ilium and ischium. Between these two sides is the sacrum which is a collection of five fused vertebrae. All the bones of the pelvis are tied together with strong ligaments which further stabilize them. The pelvis is the centre for numerous strong muscles. They attach themselves to the roughly textured and multifaceted surfaces which provide a variety of different leverage points for the muscles to work against. It is these muscles which provide the power for locomotion; the quadraceps, hamstrings, gluteus, etc.

The sacrum can be seen as a keystone in a bridge with the other bones of the pelvis acting as an arch resting upon the heads of the two femurs. This arrangement gives a broader and more stable base with the feet standing apart from each other beneath the knees and thighs. The femur and all the muscles of the thighs which help move the femur must have available a full range of movement in order to allow the femoral heads both to support the pelvis and yet move freely.

The sacrum is also the support point for the balancing of the torso pyramid upon the pelvic structure. The articulation between the sacrum and the fifth lumbar vertebrae is a crucial weight-bearing joint. In spite of the strength of the muscles and the massive size of both the pelvis and the lumbar vertebrae, it is a delicately balanced joint. It is not perfectly aligned vertically (there is a forward slant to the articulation and the lower back is structurally curved forward slightly), so attempts to make the spine straight by tucking the pelvis under the spine are both misguided and doomed to fail. Nor should the curvature be too severe. Excessive lordosis of the lumbar region or 'sway back' is equally problematic. The body is an interrelated system. If the pelvic support structure does not provide a stable support, the body will have to compensate further up the spinal column, for example, the neck, or further down the extremities, for example the knees. In fact, knee injuries often reflect restricted hip or pelvic motion. The knees, being more structurally vulnerable, give way under the repeated strain of pelvic imbalance.

Torso – the central axis
The torso is made up of the spinal column, the ribs, all the accompanying muscles, the viscera contained inside the ab-

dominal cavity and the chest cavity. The vertebrae are stacked
one on top of the other to form the spine and it is the spine more
than any other part of the skeleton which has most trouble
adjusting to the upright position. The stresses are severe and,
according to movement educator Lulu Sweigard, can usually be
attributed to one or more of the following: chronic poor alignment; inefficient or awkward movements; learned bad movement habits; improper exercise training; poor coordination;
sustained improper postural alignment due to work requirements; heavy work; or constant stress and arousal during
activity.

Though the spine curves posteriorly and dorsally there is a line
or axis which is considered to be the shortest distance between
the first cervical and fifth lumbar vertebrae. This spinal axis
should parallel closely the central axis of the whole body if the
alignment of the individual is good. The more this spinal axis
departs from the central axis of the body, the more you can look
for stress to produce damage and dysfunction in any of the
weight-bearing joints of the body.

One of the worst uses of language when describing the body is
the commonly accepted phrase 'rib cage'. In order to function
properly, the rib cage as a whole must be thought of as being soft
and malleable. Remember they are not holding the whole structure rigid and together, they too are suspended from the spinal
vertebrae. Proper posture will allow free movement of the ribs
during breathing and physical activity. And the functioning of
the internal organs: lungs, heart, intestines, etc, should be
undisturbed during physical activity. They are suspended from
the spine which, while flexible, should be relatively stable
during movement.

Neck and head – orientation
The head contains most of the teleceptors: the eyes, nose and
ears which help us orient ourselves in our environment. It is
essential that it be free to move in as wide a range as possible.
The head rests, almost floats, on top of the atlas vertebra, the
first of the seven cervical vertebrae. These have a far greater
range of movement than any of the other spinal vertebrae,
allowing an extended rotation of the head about the spinal axis.

The head can be considered to be the top of the three upside-
down pyramids, balanced on the broad base of the shoulder

girdle: the ribs, sternum, clavicles and scapulae. In order to keep the head delicately balanced on the top of the spine it is supported by a number of muscles which range round it like guy wires on a tent pole. Again, attempts to force the alignment of the head over the spine by pulling the chin in and shoving the chest forward can only result in unnecessary muscular strain or chronically rigid torso and spinal conditions with the resultant restrictions in mobility.

Suspension structure

Four-legged animals have always relied on a 'ridgepole' structure for their anti-gravity function. The spine, with all of the muscles, ribs, internal organs attached to it, is hung parallel to the ground between the four legs which provide a stable and strong base. In our upright human position, however, in order to organize the weight around a now vertical 'tent pole' structure (the upright spine) we have to hang everything from it. And because of our peculiar but unavoidable history as an animal, almost everything seems to be hanging from the front. The result is what can be called a suspension/compression structure. Everything in front is suspended from the spine and the weight of this suspension is transmitted down through the spine and eventually to the ground. It's like a crane in which the boom is hanging out away from the central support structure but the weight is carried up to the top of the central structure where it then runs down the back side to the base. The suspension weight in the front is balanced by the compression forces down the back.

It is important when focusing on the movements in any system of exercise or physical training to be aware that functionally the pelvis and lower extremities are the source of most of our locomotive power, and the head, all of its teleceptors, the shoulder girdle and the upper extremities must be as free as possible to utilize their fine motor control, differentiation and skills. Attention needs to be placed in *both* regions and we should be as familiar with the geography of the pelvis: ilium, ischium, sacrum, iliapsoas, iliacus, quadraceps and hamstrings, as we are of the shoulder girdle, sternum, clavicle, scapula and the deltoids, pectorals, and so forth. Remember you do not have to hold your shoulders for them to function properly. Rather they need to be allowed to be 'hung from above'. It is essentially faulty postural thinking to lift your chest up or push it forward. Rather you need to cultivate a circular process, thinking gently up the front of the body while thinking down the back at the same time.

The mechanics of it all

Now that we have some idea of how the body manages to stack itself so precariously up around a narrow central axis, it is time to ask the fundamental question: Why bother?

At first glance, in terms of mechanics, it is questionable that there is any advantage to it. Four-legged locomotion seems much more reliable: quadrapeds can run faster, are stronger on their feet, are closer to the ground, can jump further relative to body size, and can learn to stand much more rapidly than humans. In fact new-born calves, sheep, etc, can stand almost at birth. In addition, it would seem that even four-legged creatures like the squirrel can sit and free their forward legs for use to grasp and manipulate; on the other hand, gorillas and chimpanzees, which we think of as 'upright', run on all fours. What is so special about our upright posture?

A small moment of inertia
There is, at least, one advantage which seems to directly result from our erect posture: humans have the smallest *moment of inertia* of any creature. The moment of inertia, a characteristic of all objects, identifies the amount of energy it takes to rotate an object around its central axis. The further the mass of the object is removed from the central axis, the more energy it will take to move that mass around the axis or, for that matter, stop the movement or change its direction.

We can see this with figure skaters easily enough. When performing a spin, the skater will often start with his or her arms and perhaps one leg also extended. As the arms and legs are drawn in closer and closer to the body, the rotation increases faster and faster until the features of the skater are a blur. The same amount of energy is being used but the result is much faster and frequent rotations about the central axis as the moment of inertia is decreased by bringing the mass (arms and legs) in closer to the central axis of the body. Another way to think of it is to consider how little energy and time it takes us to turn round 360 degrees compared with the effort of a dog or horse.

High potential energy

There is however a further advantage of our upright posture. By stacking up the body parts, one on top of the other, we also achieve a high degree of *potential energy*. In other words, simply by getting so much of our body weight up high over a narrow base and located close to the central axis of the body, we can make sudden changes of direction, movement and effort without having to first get the body in position to act. It's like pounding in a stake with a sledge hammer. If you lift the sledge hammer over your head you don't have to exert nearly the same force to do the work as you would wielding it from waist level. Similarly, because our centre of gravity is so high off the ground, we can perform many actions like walking, jumping, pushing, pulling, etc without having first to get our body up off the ground.

So not only does our unique posture provide us with the ability to turn, change direction, and generally move in a wide variety of ways, but also our high potential energy allows us to perform many of these activities without having first to prepare for them.

An unstable equilibrium

But posture is not a fixed position. The human body is designed to move, not stand rigid. We have all read of guardsmen fainting because they try to stand for hours on end without so much as twitching a whisker. Any of us who have watched a Wimbledon match from the standing room part of the Centre Court, a football match from the stands, or a golf tournament from the eighteenth hole as players finish one after another, know just how strenuous it is to stand still and do nothing.

Our body parts, one stacked on another, are maintained in an equilibrium, but because the centre of gravity is so high, it is an unstable equilibrium. You become more stable as you lower your centre of gravity, and more unstable as you raise it. Standing and lying down flat represent these two extremes.

Between these positions are varying degrees of stability and instability.

Depending upon the sport or activity you pursue, you will want to move closer to a stable or unstable equilibrium. Martial arts often emphasize a lowering of the centre of gravity in order to maintain a more stable equilibrium. Even so, you will notice that the upper body is still held high and erect so as to maintain as much potential energy while still sustaining a stable position. Classical ballet often requires a high centre of gravity position – for example the standing on points so that all movements from such a position seem to be effortless and elegant in their ease precisely because there is so much potential energy available. The wobbles, fluffs, and shakes which afflict even international ballet dancers are the consequences of a very unstable high centre of gravity which accompanies their low moment of inertia and are often caused by minuscule imbalances in the equilibrium.

Good posture, to define it again then, could be said to be the use of our body which maintains our small moment of inertia and high potential energy while sustaining our bodies in an unstable equilibrium with minimum effort. The result is efficient, effortless movement.

Posture in daily life

Proper posture involves the delicate balancing of opposing forces; the extensors opening the joints out and drawing the body erect and the flexors closing the joints and drawing the extremities in. While many of the extensor muscles which act as postural muscles are 'tied into' their anti-gravity reflexes, the flexors are organized by neurological patterns which are more the product of learned experience. As a result, it is often easier to change bad postural patterns through working with the flexors which have a higher percentage of learned (if unconscious) habits. But this should be a harmonious process, not a tug-of-war. Proper posture is not produced by using flexors to lengthen extensors which may be over-contracted through incorrect use: for example, strengthening the abdominals in order to stretch the erector spinae of the lower back in order to correct low back sway. The whole process of adjusting posture is a gradual gentle collaboration with the body in which chronic patterns are released by consciously changing the muscle tonus of the hypercontracted muscles. This involves slow and gentle movements, relaxation techniques, movement awareness techniques and in general cooperation with your control system through improving your neuromuscular coordination.

Breathing
Breathing is one of the key ways of creating change in habitual postural patterns which are inefficient or misaligned. Breathing takes place in the lungs, but as discussed in the chapter on the energy system, it is really the diaphragm and muscles of the rib cage which perform the actual pumping action in the lungs. Bad posture will inevitably affect the functioning of the diaphragm. If the ribs are not hanging freely, suspended from the spine, then the intercostal muscles which move them must perform extra work to hold the ribs in place. Or, as is often the case, they are held rigid in order to conform to misguided conceptions of strength, stability and 'manliness'. This in turn affects the functioning of the diaphragm. In addition, if the pelvis is not positioned properly under the spine so as to support the weight of the upper body, the diaphragm may start to perform the function of the iliopsoas muscles, levator ani, quadratus, and abdominals, that is, stabilizing the pelvis beneath the fifth lumbar vertebra. In fact it should be the other way around. These muscles and associated other muscles should not only stabilize the pelvis but should be able indirectly to assist the diaphragm in the breathing process.

Through constant arousal or excitation, our breathing apparatus becomes keyed up for performance. The fight or flight response, when it is over-activated, will maintain the organism in a constant state of preparation. It is precisely this subliminal state of preparation (valuable for performing a task, playing a sport, defending oneself, etc) which will begin to interfere with natural breathing, if there is no opportunity to release this unconscious tension. Most of us need to learn how to let go, stop, relax, and breath out! *Expiration*, not inspiration, is the key to releasing the unconscious holding patterns in bad posture. By voluntarily letting go of the holding patterns in the flexors of the body in conjunction with exhalation we can free the anti-gravity mechanisms which maintain our upright posture without strain. In addition, learning to interrupt the muscular patterns which respond to the fight or flight response will also help the body to maintain its upward alignment without effort. And it is the effortlessness of our *functioning* whether standing, running, swimming, or dancing, which is the true reflection of correct posture.

Volitional control

Moshe Feldenkrais gives four criteria for what he calls 'coordinated, well learned action'. They are:

Absence of effort   Whether you are talking about a judo master, a downhill skier, a dancer, a yoga adept or weightlifter, correct use of the body in the performance of their skill will inevitably look like an easy, controlled and effortless movement. Interrupted breathing, straining, spinal stress, rigidity, will all show up in movement which involves poor use of the self.

Absence of resistance   By this we mean that the body is not fighting itself as it performs an action. Internal resistance to the movement and hence excess effort and unnecessary stress are minimalized.

Reversibility   This, perhaps unfamiliar, idea is the litmus test of correct movement: The ability to stop a movement at any point and reverse it indicates both a conscious neuromuscular control over the movement and appropriate postural alignment and balance. We should be *moving* from one position to another *not falling* into it. The exception to this guideline is, of course, movements which involve jumping or consciously controlled falling (as in dance).

Uninterrupted breathing   Movement patterns which evoke holding of the breath unnecessarily for sustained periods or erratic breathing patterns are almost certainly the product of muscle groups being held unconsciously in the chest, abdomen, throat and neck. Breathing should be able to progress with as much regularity as possible during exercise which works with good posture.

All four of the above guidelines involve a high degree of voluntary control over the functioning of the body. In learning correct posture we are really learning how voluntarily to control or change unconscious habits and patterns of movements.

Emotional patterns of posture

Stopping unnecessary fight or flight arousal and interrupting unconscious inhalation or unconscious holding of the breath are ways of changing total body patterns which contribute to bad posture. Learning to recognize the anxiety creating situations and individuals which contribute to these muscular states is another way of reducing bad posture. Most of these muscular patterns have emotional bases, learned experiences with parents, family, friends, co-workers. These emotional patterns maintain the bad posture by contributing to the unnecessary arousal which causes the bad habits. Interrupting emotional responses is yet another way of beginning to create changes in the total pattern which contributes to posture and alignment. Physical training should help contribute to this self-knowledge rather than trying to gloss over it. Counterproductive patterns should be let go of rather than simply forced into superficial patterns which resemble some idealized stance or posture. Almost all of the muscles you can actually touch with your hands are not posture muscles. The surface muscles are usually second or third class levers which perform physical activities, move your extremities, help you run, lift things and jump. The actual postural muscles are usually first class levers attached directly to the axial skeleton. You can't usually feel them by touching the body. So, in order to train yourself in good posture, it is necessary to interrupt the unconscious but learned patterns discussed above. You can't simply 'exercise' to make your muscles stronger, in order to pull your skeleton into alignment. Rather you have to let go and let be.

Relaxation

Why include relaxation in a book about fitness and exercise? Because the ability to relax, essential to our health, is no longer automatic in our high-stress world. It is a mental/physical skill which nowadays needs to be learned and cultivated in the same way as flexibility or endurance. The motivation for learning relaxation is the health benefits which accrue. In 1975 Dr Herbert Benson, in extensive research at Harvard University, concluded that most of the diseases of the heart and brain, causing over 50 per cent of the deaths every year in the United States, are related to hypertension. In a comparison of several major relaxation systems, he discovered that *all* of them contributed to changes for the better in the levels of several key measurements of stress which have been contributory to diseases of the heart and brain. His conclusions were simple and unavoidable: relaxation improves your health.

On the other side of the Atlantic, Dr Johannes Schultz had been collecting extensive documentation for over 30 years proving that his Autogenic Training technique was effective in the treatment of disorders of the respiratory tract – asthma and hyperventilation; the circulatory system – high blood pressure and irregular heart beat; the gastro-intestinal tract – ulcers, constipation and gastritis; and the endocrine system – thyroid problems. The implications, though hard to believe, were becoming clearer and clearer: relaxation creates changes in the functioning of the body on levels which were formerly thought to be beyond the reach of the individual's will: the involuntary nervous system, the glandular system and other self-regulating systems of the body.

Part of the problem in talking about relaxation techniques is the confusion of the terms commonly used.

Tension is the result of muscular contraction. Excess tension arises when parts of the body are overworking for the effort required to do the task at hand. Sustained and unnecessary muscle contraction in the body is a manifestation of tension.

Relaxation is the reduction of tension and a movement towards homeostasis (balance) in the body. Effort and muscle tonus are usually reduced and metabolic activity in the body usually lowered.

Arousal is in many ways the opposite of relaxation. It involves a general increase in the functions of the body: heart beat, breathing, blood pressure, attention to stimuli, etc.

Anxiety is a psychological state which is usually accompanied by constrictions in the breathing and chest, tension in the gastro-intestinal area, conflict in choices which tend to lead to either pleasure or pain; it may include increased heart beat, digestive disorders and states of fear.

Stress is a situation in which the nervous system is aroused by internal and/or external 'stressors' which disrupt your homeostasis or internal balance. There is nothing wrong with stress itself and stress is reduced when homeostasis is restored (as happens during relaxation), but unrelieved stress over an extended period can result in actual breakdown of functions in the physical organism.

We all experience these different states at different times. But in order to understand the importance of relaxation we need to understand the physiological basis for these different states of relaxation, arousal, tension, etc, as well as their relationship to our autonomic nervous system.

The fight or flight response is a self-protective mechanism which mobilizes all the necessary components of the body and nervous system to protect the integrity of the organism, in this case: you. The response is primordial and can be seen in such animal reactions as a cat arching its back and hissing, the hair standing up on the back of a dog or a rabbit suddenly bolting from its frozen hiding position. This fight or flight response is orchestrated in our autonomic nervous system. If you refer back to The Control System (pages 81–92) you will remember that our nervous system is divided into two parts. The central nervous system deals with the skeletal muscle and organizes our movement. We can consciously participate in the control of this system. The second part, the peripheral nervous system has as a subdivision, the autonomic nervous system, over which we have no apparent control and which is again divided into two parts: the sympathetic and the parasympathetic. It is the sympathetic part of the autonomic nervous system which activates the physiological functions we associate with excitement, work and physical activity as well as states like stress and arousal. When the fight or flight response is stimulated by a perceived threat, the sympathetic nervous system rushes in to provide all the necessary back-up to the skeletal muscles (which your central nervous system then marshalls into action): your heart beat quickens, blood flow to the muscles increases, adrenalin is released into the blood stream, pupils dilate. 'Fight or flight' ensues and hopefully you survive to live and breed another day.

In modern-day men and women the fight or flight response is still called into action in a wide variety of situations from presenting a report to the board of directors to crossing a busy intersection, from preparing for an important tennis match to a run down a ski slope. But not all of these situations use all the potential generated by the flight or fight response. The metabolic response may be out of proportion to the event. Stress or anxiety-producing situations which threaten possible pain or discomfort often arouse the fight or flight response under conditions where we cannot spring into action and flee. You can't fight or flee when interviewing for an important job! You'd never get it. But repeated arousal of the fight or flight response in situations where it cannot be expressed, so that the build-up of arousal and tensions in the body cannot be released, leads to chronic over-arousal, stress and tension. All other considerations being equal, chronic stress is a major factor in the cause of hypertension, as well as a principal contributor to disease and illness of any sort since chronic stress also reduces the effectiveness of our immune system.

But it goes even further. Most functions of the other half of your autonomic nervous system, the parasympathetic nervous system, are directly associated with repair and regeneration. Blood flows to the central organs where it is filtered, replaced, and replenished with nutrients from the digestive system. Blood, bones and tissues are repaired, the body is restored to readiness for activity and the future demands to be made upon it. If you don't spend time in this rest and restoration cycle, toxins build up, digestion is incomplete, old cells are not replaced and overall health deteriorates. Medical specialists are now realizing that the single common factor in a wide range of diseases from colds and ulcers to kidney failure, diverticulitis and on up to strokes, heart disease and cancer, is stress. Most of us have become habituated to a constant low level of arousal. In fact, Dr Walter R. Hess, the Swiss Nobel Prize winning physiologist, suggests that we become 'ergotropically tuned' like a guitar string which is constantly sharp. Nowadays we incline toward arousal and over-stimulation even when it is not necessary, and our lives are full of stimulants that keep us that way: coffee, alcohol, cigarettes, sugar, TV, film, entertainment, etc.

Stress is addictive and easily becomes a way of life, a habit, as familiar as our well worn running shoes.

A multitude of situations in daily life contribute to over-arousal and stress. Drs Thomas Holmes and Richard Rahe, from the University of Washington Medical School, have devised a scale of typical situations which lead to stress. It includes not only job pressures and family deaths but also moving to a new home, and marriage.

A relaxation technique properly carried out helps you learn to reverse this process. You begin to control your over-aroused responses. An effective relaxation technique forms the cornerstone to physical well being and is an essential skill to learn as the counter balance to the more active movement systems discussed in this book.

There are eight factors which are instrumental in effective relaxation techniques. Not all of them are essential but most systems involve the majority of these guidelines.

1 Progression Most relaxation techniques provide some kind of progressive cues to the body. You move through a sequence of exercises which together in a session or over a period of time build up cumulatively to produce an effect.

2 Quiet environment Retreating to a quiet place and with minimal distractions is part of the preparation for relaxation. Even techniques like yoga and t'ai chi are usually done in a quiet, peaceful place. Distractions are minimized.

3 Objects to focus on A number of systems suggest you put your attention on an object. Concentration is part of relaxation and an object to focus one's attention on takes the mind away from thoughts and ideas which may disturb, arouse or cause anxiety.

4 Passive attitude Several disciplines suggest that you observe but do not engage. You watch thoughts, feelings, sensations but avoid speculating, thinking, mind wandering. You observe without judging.

5 Comfort In order to reduce anxiety to a level where you can control it, you have to be physically comfortable and secure. In the section on posture and alignment this is outlined more clearly.

6 Breathing Many relaxation techniques use breathing either as a focus for concentration or work with the breathing mechanisms (rib, diaphragm, throat, etc) to reduce anxiety levels directly. Breathing can be an interface between the central and autonomic nervous system. It directly reflects levels of arousal, tension, anxiety and stress. Changing your breathing results in changing the 'anti-relaxation' tendencies in your body.

7 Body Cues Many relaxation techniques rely heavily upon body cues. You tie subjective emotional and mental states into the physiological sensations of the body. Changing the language you use with your body changes its response.

8 Imagery particularly imagery which has a high component of sensory cues: feeling, seeing, hearing, touching, smelling, temperature, weight, colour, etc, are more powerful signals to the body than abstract words or ideas. Imaginary journeys to a pastoral scene, the seaside, down elevator shafts to a quiet, private room, trips up a mountain, etc, can all evoke a change in the physiological state of the individual.

Relaxation techniques

Progressive relaxation was developed by Dr Edmund Jacobson, a Chicago physician, psychiatrist, and the 'grandfather' of modern day relaxation techniques. First outlined in 1929 in his book *Progressive Relaxation*, it is a simple, straightforward technique with considerable empirical backing. Jacobson maintains that you cannot have emotional anxiety or stress when your body is physiologically relaxed. Anxiety causes the body to build up unexpressed arousal which remains as tension, which in turn contributes to the underground feeling of anxiety which, in turn, causes more tension and so forth in a vicious spiral. Most individuals under stress do not even realize how chronically tense their muscles are; Jacobson felt that ignorance of your body was as inexcusable as flying without any training.

The basic technique consists of a sequential tensing and releasing of muscle groups in the body, while resting in a comfortable position either lying down or sitting with back support. Training sessions are usually for several weeks and it is suggested that you practise 15 minutes twice a day. The system is 'progressive' on three levels: First, each muscle is relaxed further and further in the course of the exercise. Second, you move progressively through the major muscle groups of the body. Thirdly, you practise each day and so the effects of relaxation are cumulative, or progressive.

The relaxation response is expounded by Dr Herbert Benson in the book of the same name. It is an equally simple and effective system for developing the ability to relax. Benson maintains that just as we have a fight or flight response, we also have a relaxation response and it is as important to develop this relaxation response as it is to be able to respond rapidly to danger. In fact, just as the fight or flight response ensured our ancestors' survival, it may be that given the environmental conditions of modern man, our ability to train ourselves in the relaxation response may ensure our survival. It is possible that we may even be selecting genetically against those individuals who don't know how to relax!

The relaxation method proposed by Benson is based upon his research into the effects of the Transcendental Meditation technique (TM). The physiological changes he observed in his systematic studies at Harvard over the years were so marked, so consistent and so apparently beneficial to the health of the individuals who practised TM that he chose it as his model.

This involves sitting quietly and comfortably, eyes closed, for 15–20 minutes twice a day and silently repeating to oneself a mantra, or word, such as 'OM' or 'peace'.

Autogenic training was developed by Dr Johannes Schultz, a Berlin psychiatrist, and is a sophisticated system for inducing substantial changes in the nervous system. Schultz based his work initially on the findings of the nineteenth century physiologist and student of hypnotic states, Oskar Vogt. Schultz combined Vogt's auto-suggestions concerning warmth and heaviness (two very common sensations experienced by hypnotic subjects who were able to eliminate tension under trance) with other specific messages to the body designed to influence the autonomic nervous system and with basic techniques demonstrated to him by yoga masters.

The first stage of training involves giving yourself certain verbal commands with accompanying feelings over several weeks. The first exercise at this stage invokes the sensation of heaviness, giving verbal command to arms and legs for them to feel heavy. The second week's commands suggest that the limbs feel warm and evokes blood flow increase to the extremities. The third command, 'My heart beat is calm', normalizes cardiac activity. The fourth involves the respiratory system: 'It breathes me'. And so on through the remaining commands. Autogenic training is a graduated progression of suggestive commands to the body spread over several months. The initial phase takes 8–12 weeks. Autogenics should be practised twice a day for fifteen minutes. However, Schultz and Luthe (his co-worker) suggest that you take a few minutes several times a day, as much as a dozen times a day, to inculcate the physiological response into your nervous system.

Autogenics is clearly engaging more than just muscle relaxation. Like the simple slogans of advertising, autogenics operates on a subliminal level to induce sophisticated changes and using the simplest of commands, it slowly cultivates some kind of volitional, if still basically unconscious, control over the autonomic nervous system. A contradiction in terms? Not really. There is now increasing scientific evidence that systematic and sophisticated control of many of the formerly 'involuntary' functions in the body is possible. Relaxation is a state of mind and a state of body. There is no doubt that changing either physiological tension and arousal or psychological anxiety and stress results in an increase in relaxation and a lowering of anxiety states.

A number of movement systems can also produce a deep experience of physical and psychological relaxation. The Feldenkrais Method, yoga, t'ai-chi, the Alexander Technique, and dance release work can all lower arousal and anxiety as well as reduce counterproductive tension in the muscles of the body. Furthermore, interrupting strenuous training sessions in any sport or exercise with a brief period of relaxation using your own or recognized technique can result in increased ability to learn new skills and improve performance. It can also postpone exhaustion and reduce the risk of injuries. Relaxation is *not* watching TV, playing snooker or having a drink; neither need it be just something you only practise for 20 minutes a day at home. It is an integral part of an ongoing training programme, and should eventually become an integral part of a healthy approach to life.

Training Principles

Whatever your particular sport, exercise system, martial art or physical activity, there are basic principles which apply to increasing your performance. These principles are not laws so much as guidelines for appropriate training. By implementing them you can pursue not only the activity you practise but also complementary systems of physical training in order to enhance your performance across the board.

1 Specificity The closer the training movements parallel the kinds of physical activity you are training for, the more effective the influence of training on performance. For example, activities which require strength at specific joint angles, such as water skiing or gymnastics, will benefit most from isometric strength training which works at the same joint angles. Long distance runs are more effective training for the marathon than sprints. Tennis practice against an opponent is ultimately more effective than against a ball machine. This is one reason why seasonal changes of sporting activity require specific training for the new sport taken up. The practice of skills which appear very similar but have significant differences will not necessarily improve the neuromuscular coordination in either of them. Practising a squash swing, which requires more wrist motion than tennis, may not improve your tennis service – in fact, control system confusion between two marginally different skills can easily be detrimental to both. Similarly, classical and modern dance styles may all seem part of 'dance' to the novice but the turnout developed by ballet, for instance, will have to be unlearned for modern styles. Neuromuscular considerations like sequencing, phasing and force change even within a specific sport. As you improve your running speed from a beginner's 10 minutes a mile, the stride changes and a 4 or 6 minute pace will involve different stride characteristics than an 8 or 10 minute pace.

2 Overload This principle is particularly important for any strength training system. Overloading stimulates the physiological processes which lead to increasing the strength and size of the muscle fibres which do the work. Actual strength is governed by the intensity of the overload as well as the specific method.

In endurance training, the training sensitive zone allows you to work at a level which puts an overload on your cardiovascular system without risking damage, strain or possible heart failure.

3 Progressive resistance Particularly applicable in strength training, flexibility training and endurance training, this principle maintains that as you improve it is necessary to increase progressively the demands you are making upon your body. *In strength training*, since an overloaded muscle actually gains strength through repeated exertions, what was formerly a maximal amount of weight for a muscle group subsequently becomes easier and easier to lift. It is then necessary to increase the weight load in order to continue to make the maximal demands upon the muscles. *In endurance training*, through regular running or swimming, for example, what were previously maximal times and distances become progressively easier and easier to achieve. You must increase the distance and times in order to continue to achieve the training results. *In flexibility training*, range of movement increases through repetition of exercise and you can expect to stretch further or perform more complicated exercises in order to continue to extend your flexibility. Even in relaxation techniques the principle of progression is vital. Different stages of a relaxation programme are designed to build one upon another so that a cumulative effect is achieved in the control of arousal and excitation.

A word of caution. In all activities you will reach a level at which it becomes increasingly difficult to improve further. If you are engaged in a strenuous and demanding training programme, then it may be inappropriate to make further demands upon your body in the form of heavier weights, longer distances or increased hours of stretching exercise. Often it is invaluable to put more time and energy into pursuing increased neuromuscular coordination and skill practice. Alternatively, training in a complementary sport or activity will enhance your performance further in your chosen discipline. Proper relaxation may be the actual key to increased performance. *Avoid the overtraining syndrome* (see page 151 for overtraining warning signals).

4 Regularity Whatever training programme you take part in, regularity of participation is important. In fact, consistency in training often plays *the* key role in ultimate achievement of goals in performance. Having said that, you don't necessarily have to follow in the footsteps of the rather extraordinary British marathoner, Ron Hill, who claims to have strung together over six thousand consecutive days of training and conditioning. In some cases, like strength training, three or four training sessions a week will be enough. For yoga or endurance training you can extend that to five or six days a week without too many problems. Relaxation techniques, on the other hand, benefit from very regular and consistent practice with no restrictions on the number of days a week. You may find in general that performance and well being are enhanced by alternating one form of training with others throughout the week. A body conditioning class will complement a strength training programme or tennis matches, nicely. Aikido and skiing will be compatible. Dance and stretch classes go hand in hand.

5 Rest and recovery There is a long-standing coaching adage: 'Train, don't strain'. The balance between effective training 'to maximal effort' and safe training procedures is not easy for a professional coach to achieve, never mind the eager amateur, so it is not necessarily wise or beneficial to push yourself compulsively to the maximal levels of performance. Recovery is as important a principle as overload or specificity. Some techniques like t'ai chi or the Feldenkrais Method, in which the body is not overtaxed due to the characteristics of these movement systems, will benefit from really consistent practice. Relaxation techniques can be practised every day with no overtraining side-effects. The best guideline for the balance between training and rest seems to be that the harder you train in terms of physical effort and work accomplished, the more time that has to be allowed for rest and recovery.

6 Arrangement Exercises in any training programme should be arranged so that you get the best possible results while guarding against any damage or injury. In weight training, for example, the exercises should be arranged so that larger muscle groups are worked before smaller muscle groups. The training programme should also be organized so that different muscle groups are exercised in sequence: the overhead standing press and the bench press should not be performed one after another since they involve similar muscle groups. Stretching of the hamstrings is best followed by working with the adductors in the legs or perhaps even by working the antagonistic muscle groups such as the quadraceps. In skill learning you might want to begin with fine motor movements and differentiation of body parts before combining them into larger and grosser movement patterns. Sports which are continuous, particularly ones like running or cycling, are best practised as a whole with perhaps changes in emphasis on speed, force or phasing. In activities which consist of a number of discreet skills like tennis or ballet the different skills can be practised separately. In classical ballet training, for example, a class will progress through the repertoire of steps, moves and jumps separately before combining them into an entire dance sequence.

7 The proper training environment For some sports practising your skills in a variety of situations leads to a more substantial grounding of the skill in your control system. Skiing on a variety of terrains and in different snow conditions results in the skills being more thoroughly learned and consequently more accessible to you in the wide range of situations you might encounter on the slopes. Sparring with partners of all different shapes, sizes and abilities serves the same function in martial arts. At the same time, the atmosphere and climate of your tae kwon do, or aikido dojo, may be an essential element of the total experience so that each time you train, the regime will be consistent and familiar.

Arousal levels are also an important element of the training atmosphere. Generally, a non-threatening, supportive environment encourages learning. Finding the proper level of arousal is essential. Search out the right teacher and the right level of class so that your level of arousal is optimal for you and for the activity you are pursuing. Physical exercise and training should strike the right balance between strong demands placed upon the body which encourage it to excel beyond past limitations and the need for conscious control and direction of movement in an environment which is conducive to learning.

8   Recognition of different physical goal requirements Every physical goal requires a different approach. You may want to increase your repetitions in strength training in order to increase muscle bulk, but in skill development and neuro-muscular coordination it is vital *not* to overload the nervous system. Repetition of movement patterns and sequences must allow for integration into the controlling areas of the brain. Excess practice can lead to lack of discrimination and differentiation: you no longer know if you are training properly or not. Performance deteriorates and you begin to practise badly, or wrongly. Flexibility training deteriorates if movements are too rapid. Endurance training calls for sustained repetition of the same skill whereas improvement in posture may require constant interruption of habitual patterns. Cooperate with the physiological requirements of each training goal.

9   Don't overtrain Along with ignorance, over-enthusiasm and poor coaching, overtraining is a major contributor to injury and poor performance. Develop a healthy relationship with your body and listen to the warning signals which may be the indication of early stages of overtraining.

Warning Signals

1 A 6–12 beats per minute elevation in morning, at resting heart rate. This is perhaps the most common, easily recorded warning that the body has not totally recovered from the previous day's stresses.

2 A consistent elevation in the normal body temperature of a degree or two. Again, this physiological parameter is relatively easy to monitor, and it informs the individual of the resting state of the body.

3 A low-level, but persistent stiffness and soreness in the muscles, tendons and joints.

4 Frequent minor sore throats and colds, or development of mouth ulcers.

5 Excessive nervousness, irritability, headaches, depression, anxiety with no apparent cause.

6 Inability to sleep, rest or relax normally.

7 Nagging fatigue and general sluggishness that continues for several days.

8 Unexplained, noticeable drops in performance.

9 Disinterest in normally exciting and stimulating activities.

10 Diarrhoea or constipation.

11 Aching stomach or feeling of uneasiness in the abdomen.

12 Loss of appetite and body weight.

13 Elevated readings for nocytes (white blood cells) and atypical lymphocytes (lymph cells) in the blood count.

from 'Warning Signs and Symptoms of Overtraining and Overstress', Alfred Morris, *Sports Medicine*

PART TWO

Western Sports

Human beings have always striven towards excellence. Nowhere is this manifested more clearly than in the field of sports performance. The need to excel in physical performance is a human urge constant to all peoples of all periods throughout the world. Stories have come down to us from the earliest times of individuals and groups pitting their strength against each other or against the forces of nature.

Sport in its most primitive form derived from ritualistic enactments of the hunt or the encounter between the hunter and the forces of nature or beast. The rituals took the form of dances and ceremonies but the encounter of strength, willpower and skill was also expressed in games.

And just as the best hunter would receive the accolade of the tribe so it is the striker in a football team today who gets the cheers of the crowd. The interlinking of hunting skills and sport is still evident in the language we use, since the same skills were used to protect the tribe's territory. Phrases like 'establish a position', 'stake out one's ground', 'guard the plate', 'to dominate and defend', are common to many sports.

The most renowned athletes in the history of sport are the ancient Greeks. Many of the sagas from *The Iliad* contain accounts of sporting events, heroic feats and funeral games and it is to the Greeks that we owe the first organized games: the Olympics. The setting was at the site of the mythical contest between Zeus and Chronos to determine who would become the leader of the gods. Around 1000 BC Olympia was consecrated to Zeus (the winner) and some years later games were staged there to win his approval. The games were held every four years during which a moratorium on war and conflict was called through the land. (Would that the Olympics had such power today!)

Games were held all over Greece, reflecting the fundamental belief that the pursuit of sports as a means of bettering oneself was equal to training the mind. Body and mind were very much one in the Greek vision. Socrates emphasized the importance of physical well being and Plato maintained that gymnastic exercise was the 'twin sister' of the arts 'for the improvement of the soul'.

The Romans continued this ideal, and their adage 'mens sana in corpore sano' (a sound mind in a sound body) has enjoyed a resurgence with the current fitness boom. By AD300 there were nearly 200 public holidays and 175 of these were given over to games and spectacles to keep the masses entertained; this was one way of dealing with the large numbers of unemployed. As professionalism became the norm, athletes were less and less able to use their specialized skills for combat and war. The Roman solution to this was the gladiatorial contest. These bloodthirsty spectacles cast a shadow over the simpler athletic pursuits and much of the spirit of the Greek games was lost.

With the fall of Rome the Middle Ages brought a return to more localized and provincial forms of games and competitions. While the Greeks organized sporting competition on a national level, unparalleled until the re-emergence of the modern Olympics, the medieval diversification and rich variety of idiosyncratic pastimes formed the antecedents of most of the games we play today.

Ball games developed all over Europe: German tribes played kagels, the Irish, hurling, and the Scots, shinty. In these early Christian times playing on Sundays after church was encouraged as a form of recreation and in villages without common land the church cloisters were used. France was the origin of 'paille maille', which was brought to London by James I. The road names Pall Mall and the Mall indicate where the game was first played. While paille maille involved hitting a ball with a stick, 'la soule au pied' is the antecedent of football.

The wide gap between the classes was reflected in an equally wide difference in leisure pursuits. While the peasants played ball games and held team events, the privileged enjoyed racing, hunting and hawking. Only the wealthy could afford a horse, had rights to the finer game (such as deer) and could keep and train a hawk.

The affluent humanitarians of the Italian Renaissance revived the ideal of the scholar/athlete. In 1526 Baldassare Castiglione published *The Book of the Courtier* in which he wrote that the ideal courtier was well built and 'shapely of limb'. He should practise fencing and riding and would know how to leap, run, swim and play tennis. A few years later in England, Sir Thomas Elyot's *Book of the Governour* echoed these merits of physical education for the gentleman.

But the emergence of puritanism put a dampener on this Renaissance flowering. Luther himself approved of a limited practice of physical exercise but the extremist Calvin in Geneva denounced all sports as devilish pastimes, and football, quoits and a whole variety of ball and stick games were soon prohibited.

It was at this point that politics first entered sport, when James I issued a proclamation on 'Lawful Sports' which flew in the face of puritan doctrine. But later Cromwell enforced a widespread ban on sport and recreational pursuits. It was only with the inveterate gambler Charles II that games were allowed again in Britain. Newmarket was established and Charles brought ice skating back with him from his exile in Holland. Women started to play lawn tennis, water sports came into vogue, and swimming, rowing and later yachting were all encouraged.

The eighteenth and nineteenth centuries were to see the regularization of most of the common sports as we know them today. First came the Jockey Club in 1750. The Honourable Company of Edinburgh Golfers was established in 1744, but it was ten years later at St Andrews that the first thirteen simple rules were drawn up. And in 1787 the Marylebone Cricket Club was founded in London. James Figg started the first boxing school near Oxford road, presiding as 'Master of the Noble Art of Self Defence', and it was a student of his, Jack Broughton, who introduced the rules which revolutionized boxing, such as no hitting below the belt or when a man is down.

The regulating bodies that were founded throughout the sporting world arose in response to the increasing popular interest in sport. The industrial revolution heralded the beginning of mass leisure, which brought both increased participation in sporting activities and increased spectators.

The nineteenth century saw the explosion of team sports, and football took over as the pre-eminent sport of the general public. At first every village and school played according to its own rules and on different pitches, until in 1863 a number of London clubs formed the Football Association, laying down national rules for the game which came to be called soccer (after Assoc. Football). This, in turn, led to the establishment of the Rugby Football Union in 1871, which formulated its own rules for the type of football traditionally played at Rugby School. Football was promulgated far and wide and by the end of the century it had shifted from being an upper-class game to one of the most generally popular team sports, played throughout Europe, South America, Australia and New Zealand.

Cricket remained a sport of the privileged classes and its slower pace did not attract the same crowd enthusiasm as football. In America baseball swept the states and became the national pastime of unprecedented standing. Tennis had set up regulations and, in 1877, the All England Croquet Club added tennis to its name and sponsored the first Wimbledon tennis championships. Snow skiing gained in popularity and developed from pragmatic beginnings into a chic pastime. In Canada ice skating and ice hockey were formalized and developed. Athletic clubs began to form, gymnasia were built and indoor sports flourished. Basketball was invented, squash as well. By the end of the 19th century sport was transformed from the pursuit of the leisured or diversions for the working classes into seriously competitive activities with regulating bodies and established rules which applied not only at home but internationally.

Technological advances made the development of port in the twentieth century overwhelming. Equipment became more sophisticated and consistent. Sewing machines made costumes affordable and incandescent lighting made indoor competition possible in the evenings after work. Sport was now affordable to the ordinary working people, and the rise in public transport took spectators further afield to matches.

The 1890s saw the revival of the Olympic tradition. Although the burgeoning of sport centred on Victorian England, it was a Frenchman, Baron Pierre de Coubertin, who lobbied around the world for a reintroduction of the Olympics. The first was finally held in 1896 in Greece. It was a modest affair: 200 athletes from twelve different countries joined 200 Greek athletes. Strictly for men only, the events excluded the chariot race and pancrateon of the original Olympics and added fencing, high jump, pole vault, hurdles, weight lifting, gymnastics, tennis, swimming and cycling. It was to be held every four years and rotate from city to city and nation to nation.

It took many years of determination on their part before women were finally included in the games in 1928. Baron de Coubertin had blocked their entry successfully for years, reasoning that women athletes were 'against the laws of nature', and 'the most inaesthetic sight human eyes could contemplate'. But the following Olympics in 1932 saw the emergence of one of the all-time great women athletes. American Mildred 'Babe' Didrikson could run, throw, leap, swim, ride and hit or kick almost anything. When asked by a condescending male reporter if there was any game she did not play, she replied, after considering a moment: 'Yeah . . .dolls'. She won two gold medals and one silver, shattering records in the javelin and 80 metres hurdles. (Women were limited to a choice of three out of the five events open to them.)

International politics entered sport with a bang in 1936 when Hitler stage-managed the Berlin Olympics for the aggrandizement of the Third Reich, organizing huge military parades and selecting which athletes' hands he shook, avoiding congratulating the great Jesse Owens or any of the other black athletes. It was a nice irony that Jesse Owens should emerge as a major contestant on the international scene during the 1936 Olympics, flaunting Nazi Germany's claims to Aryan supremacy by winning four gold medals.

Following their devastation in the Second World War, the Russians emerged in force in the 1952 Olympics to stun the world by winning 71 medals, only five short of the USA's 76. The Soviet Union and the Eastern European countries have continued to allocate vast resources for the furtherance of sporting excellence, providing top quality facilities for all to enjoy, thereby ensuring the fostering of athletic potential at all levels and the cultivation of an elite to reckon with on the international scene.

Barriers were being broken at all levels. Not only were times and records tumbling but also racial and male-female barriers were giving way, in the recognition at last of skill, talent and training over old prejudices. But there were problems born out of this vastly increased interest in sport.

Since the First World War, when sports news first provided a much needed antidote to the unrelieved gloom and destruction of the years of war reporting, the media has seen in sport a rich source of exploitable material. Sport began to have 'stars', whose share of the limelight rivalled that of the early film stars. To the kudos of being a supreme sportsman, a winner, were added mass public adulation – and money.

As sport became big business the new breed of professional athletes flourished. Increased revenues from gate attendances and commercial sponsorship allowed former 'amateur' athletes to become professional and to pursue excellence in their sport without the need to earn a living alongside their athletic training. Professional and amateur circuits grew side by side.

Widespread commercialization of sport accompanied the growth of television coverage. Bjorn Borg came to epitomize the marriage of physical excellence and commercial acumen in his not-so-subtle sponsorship of sporting goods, winning the 1977 men's final at Wimbledon in a panoply of stickers advertising everything from sportswear to airlines. This kind of endorsement netted Borg nearly 2 million dollars a year. The TV rights to the 1988 Seoul Olympic games were purchased in the USA by NBC TV for $300 million.

The 1980s have seen the advent of the 'professional' amateur. To keep up with the state sponsorship of athletes in the Eastern bloc, national associations in the West provide the vehicle whereby members retain their amateur status by having their sizeable commercial endorsement fees paid into trust funds until such time as they 'retire' from their amateur status.

After the news pages, sport competes only with finance for the widest coverage in the papers. There are now more sports magazines on the news-stands than any other variety. Even the fashion industry has aped the style of sports people for some time now, to the point where names like Nike and Adidas are not only big business but fashion chic as well.

But for all its commercialism, occasional tarnished reputation, its bad sports and prima donnas, sport still holds a pre-eminent place for us as a measurement of physical excellence, of beauty in form and action, of team spirit and synergistic performance. It continues to uplift more people than almost any other activity, provides the potential for growth and achievement for a wider range of people than any other activity, and continues to expand to reaches certainly never fathomed by the early ball players, the Greek Olympians or the Roman emperors.

The 'sport for everyone' explosion of the last few decades has left us with a multitude of options and confused as to the choices. This section of the book is not meant to provide even a partial glossary of the sports practised today. Rather we have chosen to approach it by looking at a selection of the most commonly practised sports which represent the typical range of exercise offered.

Our choice of sports was influenced by availability to the average individual and level of popularity. So we include alpine skiing, despite its specialised nature, because it has enjoyed such a remarkable popular boom. It also differs markedly from cross-country skiing in the demands it makes on the body, so we include both for comparison.

Running, swimming, cycling and cross-country skiing all offer forms of endurance conditioning, but are completely different in terms of skills, technique and environment. On the other hand, tennis, squash and badminton are all racquet sports and while the requirements in terms of technique differ somewhat, we have settled on tennis as a representative model.

We have chosen football and volleyball as the models for team sports. Field hockey parallels football as a field sport in the physical demands it makes, but not in its popularity. Volleyball has risen to become one of the most popular women's team sports and is our representative indoor court game.

Our selection excludes, however, such sports as scuba diving, sailing, netball, basketball, bowling, fencing, horse riding, cricket, croquet, water-skiing and many other much loved and enlivening activities, some because they are object – rather than body – orientated, some because they have a minority following and others because they are refined versions of sports we do discuss. This should in no way discourage you from exploring the full range of sport but rather, by giving you an outline of fundamental principles, encourage you to develop your own personal training programme or enjoyment of a variety of different sports. We believe that the satisfaction you then derive from your chosen activity will be all the greater. This is the spirit of Stage Two Fitness.

Running

Over the last decade running has become big news. More money has been made from running than from any other sporting pastime. The plethora of running magazines, running gear, running clinics, etc, has caught the imagination of the individual and filled the wallet of many a businessman. The current hype in the popular press and commercial sector may be riding on the health benefits (or hazards), on the controversial 'runners' high', the metaphysics of the long distance runner and the Zen of running, but there is a more elemental consideration which makes running the Everyman sport: anyone can do it!

With walking, running has the lowest barrier to entry of an aerobic sport. You can trot, jog, run long slow distances or pile up five-minute miles in preparation for the marathon – all of this constitutes running. Everyone, with the exception of the physically handicapped, has run often during the course of their life, hence everyone already has the minimal requisite skill to run. You don't need any special equipment other than a pair of running shoes and you don't have to fly to St Moritz to run either. You can run in your own street, the nearby park, in your back garden, or, as in the case of one New York woman who was preparing for the marathon and could only run at night, but was afraid to venture out at dark, on your terrace. (She ran for a 5-mile circle in one direction and then an equal distance in the other to balance the training of both sides).

In the ancient Olympics there was one competition for each sport but three for running: 200 metres, 400 metres, and 4800 metres. However, it took the reintroduction of the Olympics in the nineteenth century and the expansion of the range of competitions for running to capture the imagination of the modern day spectator. A 100 metre sprint was added to the 200 and 400 metres and 400 metre relays were introduced, while the mile became a standard fixture. And of course the marathon, not a part of the original Olympics, became a favourite of the modern Games. Included in the first modern Olympics in 1896, at the insistence of the Greeks, it was won by an unknown Greek shepherd, Spiridon Loues, from the tiny village of Marousi. It was the first race he had ever run, and the last – a true amateur!

Women began to make their way in track and field events only in the 1920s, and with much determination on their part against a hostile male officialdom.

Running is a history of firsts and broken barriers. We encounter legendary figures like Jesse Owens, who in a single day at the 1936 Berlin Olympics won three of his four gold medals. Another legendary figure is Roger Bannister, who as a young medical student registered a 3.59.4 minute mile at the Iffley Road track in Oxford on 6 May 1954, thereby breaking the four minute mile. It was hailed by the press around the world as a breakthrough of major importance.

The marathon has become an epic event all over the world, from Boston to Tokyo, with tens of thousands of ordinary people competing and, in so far as they stay the course, winning.

But despite all the media attention running still ranks behind tennis, cycling, football and volleyball in the popularity rankings in most countries. Nonetheless, with cross-country skiing, swimming and rowing, running is one of the best training systems for your heart and lungs. Distance running expands and preloads the pumping chamber of the heart, and lung sizes are larger in competitive runners than in most other sportspeople (cross-country skiing being an obvious exception). At the level of highest demand (near the end of a long distance race or in a 400 or 800 metre race) top runners can exchange over 200 litres of air per minute and their VO_2Max is very high. In addition, the anaerobic threshold is higher in top level runners. For example, Frank Shorter, the marathoner, may have a lower VO_2Max than the 5000 metre record holder, Steve Perfontaine, but their time was the same over a three mile course because Shorter was able to utilize a higher percentage of his VO_2Max before reaching his anaerobic threshold.

The range of skills required in running is minimal. No other sport produces effective training results with so little input in terms of skill learning. Once you have achieved a certain level of cardiovascular fitness and brought your time down to a level you can stabilize at, the challenge becomes to improve your stride rate and length. Our running style is in large part a function of body shape: width of hips, length of thigh bones, knock-knees, etc. But learn a good, economical stride from the start, since it is hard to change movement patterns once they become established.

As running has become more and more popular the different

levels of competition available has increased: the 400 metre, the one mile, the 10 kilometre, the marathon, and even the ultra-marathon (100 miles). In addition there are more variations on running, embracing activities to suit every individual: cross-country or road races, orienteering, which combines running with map reading and quick thinking, fun runs relays, single sex, mixed and children's events. Remember that we are all different in our genetic makeup, with different mixes of heart and lung sizes, fast and slow twitch muscles, fat, bone and muscle ratios. All this affects performance and hence satisfaction not only in the sport you choose, but also in the level at which you choose to pursue it. So, if you find that marathons wipe you out don't abandon running but try out a jogging or cross-country club as this might suit your needs, personality and goals far better.

Running has certain inherent shortcomings as a primary conditioning system. The principal one is that it is limited in the muscles it trains: strengthening the back of the legs (hamstrings and calves), strengthening somewhat the buttocks, slight strengthening of the fronts of the legs (quadriceps) while contributing very little to upper body conditioning. Secondly it is one of the worst sports for flexibility. Unless you compete at top levels, you simply don't need to be very supple for the longer runs. Running chronically shortens the hamstrings and the muscles of the lower back which can lead to lower back lordosis (sway back).

Injuries are the plague of runners. With the limited range of movement of joints and the prodigious demand placed on the feet and knees it is little wonder that injury books, runners' guides and injury clinics have boomed over the last decade. The most common running injuries are achilles tendinitis, ankle sprains, runners' knee, back pain, shin splints. These can be caused by anything from an awkward stride, bad terrain, poor shoes, gaining weight, adding distance, increasing speed, to trying to avoid fellow runners. So cultivate your awareness – running is not as simple a sport as it at first appears.

Following on from this, running is not very good for posture. The sway back in particular which can cause a misalignment of the pelvis beneath the lumbar vertebrae leading to back pain, and the discrepancy between upper and lower body strength creates all sorts of alignment problems.

Because of the potential for injuries due to unbalanced demands upon the body, running should always be accompanied by some other activity like swimming, weight training or another sport for upper body conditioning, and a flexibility programme, like yoga or stretch classes, for the lower limbs and all-round suppleness. An alternative might be an awareness technique, like the Alexander Technique, or a gentle martial art like t'ai chi ch'uan.

Having given these warnings, there is no doubt that running answers some deep personal needs in individuals, which keep them at it despite the apparent drawbacks and simplicity (to outsiders, boredom) of the sport. At its simplest level running is an undisputed contributor to all-round health and well being. It is a sociable sport for those who want this, with clubs abounding and nearly always a friendly co-runner to support you in that final stretch. Equally there are those who derive immense pleasure from running alone, with no responsibilities to anyone but themselves. Some enjoy the physical exertion, others like the silence and sense of being a part of nature, right out in there with the wind, rain or whatever the weather brings. Running has its mystics and its pragmatists. The very simplicity of the sport makes achievement a daily and tangible thing, and while not high in the creativity stakes, the possibilities it offers for self-mastery and autonomy are obvious. Finally, there are many stories from regular runners, in particular long distance, describing the unique experience of going beyond the pain barrier, the aches and the shortness of breath and finding an almost trance-like or meditative state. For some this is a transcendent experience, for others it brings them to a sense of unity with their surroundings and the world.

Walking

Walking used to be a part of every person's life – a natural and unconscious daily conditioning programme. Today, despite the joggers and runners, we drive to work, take the bus two stops, take escalators and elevators, shop with the car and use it to visit friends a few blocks away. A sedentary lifestyle has been cultivated as a reflection of affluence and walking came to be viewed as a time-waster. A 15 minute walk is considered an effort by many.

However, walking is still listed as the most popular physical pastime: both the gentle country walk and the more serious hill walks enjoy a large following in Britain. Ramblers clubs abound, hill climbing, orienteering, hiking and many more opportunities for organized walking make for endless variety. And it is always possible to find an organization to support you at the level at which you wish to walk. Even at a spontaneous and irregular level walking can be one of the most enjoyable of physical activities.

The tendency since the running boom has been to relegate walking to the status of poor cousin of the more glamorous sport. But not many are aware that walking is an excellent cardiovascular conditioner. It burns energy at a substantial rate: while the average swimming or running pace burns 300 calories in 30 minutes, 40–45 minutes of brisk walking will utilize the same amount. And it is clearly a far safer exercise form for the person with a heart condition or recovering from illness or surgery than plunging straight into something more vigorous. We are not talking about the gentle stroll or saunter but walking at a sturdy pace: about 3 miles per hour which translates into roughly 1 mile in 20 minutes, for 20–40 minutes at least four times a week. Walking can safely be practised as an exercise form every day, since it does not have the stressful effect on joints or muscles of running.

Walking will improve the oxygen carrying capacity of your lungs and the ability of your circulatory system and heart to pump blood through the body. As already said, the pace must be such, and maintained for long enough, to provide this aerobic conditioning. The 3 mile per hour pace is an average speed. You will find the right pace for your own level of fitness. If you choose more hilly terrain then you can increase the conditioning effect. High speeds are attained by competitive walkers, a sport fast gaining in popularity, which is very different from recreational walking in its use of particular striding techniques and special equipment.

As an experience – physical and emotional – walking can be entirely different from jogging and running. The slower pace and natural body movement allow you to forget your body and observe your surroundings more acutely or, alternatively, to focus on your inner thoughts, attaining, as some testify, a meditative state of mind and body, a harmony and quiet sense of well being that many do not achieve in running due to the stress of the effort they are making. The list of famous and great people throughout the ages who have taken a daily constitutional and swear by its benefits is endless, embracing such opposites as Ramsay MacDonald and the spiritual teacher Krishnamurti. Some say that their walk is a time of inspiration and clear thinking: others, like Krishnamurti, claim that not a thought passes through and their mind is entirely quiet, watching, aware. You can be a part of your environment when walking in a way not offered by sports that force you to focus on technique or effort.

Walking demands nothing in the way of equipment except a good pair of shoes or boots. (But you do have the option to get into the specialist gear, like plus fours, if you move on to more sophisticated levels of activity like hill walking.) Walking calms the mind and lifts the spirit – especially if you are working all day in an indoor job. The shot of fresh air and simple movement is a wonderful tonic and available to each and every one of us. But particularly for those who feel they are beyond the age or inclination for more aggressive or competitive activities, and for those who can't fit in training schedules to a busy work life, then walking is the answer.

Swimming

Swimming is undoubtedly one of the best all-round forms of exercise available. It is recommended for sufferers of arthritis, stroke patients, heart attack patients, paraplegics and the overweight. There is almost no age limit: swimming can start from birth and continue on into old age. Individuals of all levels of physical ability and fitness can learn to swim.

Swimming has always been a recreational sport wherever climate has permitted, but until this century its popularity as a competitive sport has been limited due to the cost of building and maintaining a pool, and the minimum appeal to the spectator. In the early 1920s two totally different social phenomena completely changed the availability and social perspective of swimming. One was the YMCA. As a part of its confirmed belief in 'a healthy mind in a healthy body', the Young Men's

Christian Association began to build swimming pools in the centre of cities so that youngsters could have the opportunity to move and exercise in what was an otherwise arid urban landscape.

The second factor was the emergence of Hollywood in the 1920s and 30s as the major new trend setter. Any star worth mentioning had to have a swimming pool, whether it was used or not. The warm climate meant that the pools were open and used all the year round. Middle class families aped the stars, and a whole generation of kids grew up living in the water of the pool or the seaside. On the screen, Johnny Weissmuller of Tarzan fame was able to turn his Olympic Gold in swimming into lucrative Hollywood contracts. Esther Williams likewise brought the pool to the Busby Berkeley stage setting, the precedent for synchronized swimming.

But swimming as a 'people's sport' really emerged in the 1968 and 1972 Olympics when first Don Schollander with his five gold medals and subsequently Mark Spitz with his seven golds burst upon the international sports scene. These smiling, crew-cut, smooth limbed, nearly-naked, all-American Adonises captured the imagination of the world. Now, in the 1980s, West Germany, East Germany, Australia and England are all challenging new world records and producing new swimming marvels. Meanwhile swimming has rapidly grown to become the major alternative to running as an aerobic conditioner amongst the exercising public. It is now even possible to do body conditioning and aerobic exercises, adapted to take place in the pool. The danger of impact injury to joints is avoided and the resistance of the water increases the training effect. Swimming requires almost no equipment: just a suit, and, if you wish, some goggles and earplugs. It is easily learned and you can swim indoors, outdoors in freshwater lakes and rivers, or in the sea. You can swim for leisure and fun with no concern for training or conditioning. You can swim short distances, an hour a day or even in long distance competitive swims. But swimming in a pool for conditioning is a lonely occupation. You don't really even have the opportunity to chat or gossip with a friend as you do in running or cycling, so the motivation for those repeated pool lengths must lie elsewhere. Bear this in mind if social support is a must in your exercise programme.

Along with running, cross-country skiing and bicycling,

swimming is an exceptionally good aerobic conditioner. But, unlike cross-country skiing you don't need particularly good technique to be able to maintain yourself within the conditioning zone and unlike running and cycling, which are primarily lower body sports, swimming employs many of the major muscle groups of the body. Most of these muscle groups are used in the body equally on both sides and front and back. The lungs and cardiovascular system are well and truly cultivated: a competitively trained 15-year-old swimmer can develop a heart and lung capacity equal to that of a first class adult marathon runner. Along with a high aerobic capacity comes a high anaerobic threshold, the result of having to supply oxygenated blood to a large number of muscles rather than the more limited demands of, for example, cycling.

When monitoring your heartbeat to maintain your conditioning effect within your training sensitive zone in swimming, subtract 13 from your age-predicted maximum heart rate. If you are 30 years old and wish to train at the 70 per cent threshold level, use the following formula: $((220-30)-13 \times 70\%$.

Swimming is good for posture and alignment because of the equal distribution of use made upon the body, although tension can build up in the neck and shoulder muscles during sustained breaststroke. In addition the support of the water reduces the needs for the anti-gravity muscles to operate and so helps cut through the deep seated postural reflexes which make it so difficult consciously to change bad postural habits. Flexibility is more easily maintained. Arms, shoulder and neck are all taken through a wide but gentle range of motion. Furthermore, because there is no impact between feet and the ground, there is little chance of the stress injuries common in running or soccer. Elite or long distance swimmers who may swim up to 10,000 metres a day can develop frayed muscles and tendinitis, but these are an unlikely possibility for the average swimmer.

A good swimmer does not necessarily have to have fine motor control, or the neuromuscular coordination of an Alpine skier or a tennis player. The skills which are essential are multi-limb coordination and good control over gross body movements. It is difficult to learn a stroke in parts: swimming tends to be an all-or-nothing process. The swimmer's basic stroke is his entire repertoire and in order to perfect it competitive swimmers will put in hours and hours of training, repeating the same fundamental movement pattern. In order to train at competitive level high motivation is required to overcome the pain and boredom of such repetitive training. For the average individual who wants to keep fit anything from an hour a day to as little as half an hour 3 or 4 times a week, depending on your present level of fitness and your commitment, will produce good results.

Another dimension talked about by regular swimmers is the contact that one makes with oneself. There is a sense of unity with yourself and the water which settles over a swimmer after the first few laps of the pool, enhanced by the cocoon-like isolation from anything except your immediate watery environment. The rhythm and ease of the swimming stroke also seems to promote a deep sense of relaxation which emerges after a gentle but consistent swim.

Swimming remains one of the best all-round exercise forms available with low cost, low injury risks, easy acquisition of the skill and excellent health benefits: it is a safe bet as a training activity in itself and as a complement to sports like soccer and volleyball as well as providing a conditioning programme for cross-country skiing.

Cycling

The early 1800s saw well-to-do English, French and German eccentrics experimenting with an extraordinary range of peculiar contraptions which were the early antecedents of the modern-day bicycle. By the 1860s the bicycle had evolved into a machine consisting of an iron frame with huge front wheels and tiny back wheels, pedals and a steering mechanism, rubber tyres and sprockets and chains. But in the 1890s the pneumatic tyre, patented by John Boyd Dunlop in Belfast, and the detachable tyre and inner tube developed by the Parisian Edouard Michelin, made the bicycle comfortable as well as functional.

It was soon discovered that a good deal of strength and stamina was required to ride a bicycle and inevitably competitive cycling was born. Henri Desgranges, the editor of *L'Auto*, a French sports paper, founded the Tour de France in 1903. A six-stage race over 1500 miles, it was eventually expanded to include routes through the Alps and then the Pyrenees. 1909 saw the launch of the Giro d'Italia and the Tour de Flandres was established in 1913. Tours sprang up all over the Continent and cycling began to take on the passion characteristic of the epic races which annually obsess the national psyche of countries like France and Italy. And as competitive cycling has come into its own we have seen the burgeoning not only of road racing but time trialists, criterium and track pursuit specialists as well as team track competitions. Cycles vary: the springy low wheelbase touring cycle; the stiff short wheelbase track cycle and now even the tough broad and knobbly tyred BMX open terrain bike. They all appeal to different mentalities and different situations.

Nowadays high tech has taken over cycling. Chrome and molybdenum frames, sophisticated gearing, alloy crank sets, narrow-gauged 240 gram tyres all add up to sophisticated and increasingly expensive machines. The space age cycles first seen in action at the 1984 USA Olympic men's track pursuit events are rumoured to have each cost tens of thousands of dollars.

Cycling, in the same way as running, can be broken down into sprint, middle and long distance races. The track pursuit cyclist will need a high percentage of fast twitch fibres in his powerful leg muscles to allow a high pedalling cadence (up to 120RPMs). The time trialist, on the other hand, generally requires as much endurance fibre as possible. He must achieve an optimal speed and maintain it for anything up to 24 hours, with as little variance as possible, approaching but not exceeding his anaerobic threshold. Criterium racing falls somewhere between the two, staying in the pack and allowing for periodic bursts of speed to make a break or catch up with another cyclist.

Road racing is closest to the cycling of the average person and is primarly an endurance sport with some strength ability in order to climb hills, change pedalling cadence, accelerate with competitors, etc. Tour de France competitors generally have a 70/30 ratio of slow twitch/fast twitch fibres in their leg muscles.

A large heart and lungs go with the sport. Cycling is an excellent cardiovascular conditioner and is often recommended for weight control since it produces the same cardiovascular training effect as swimming or running. But due to the efficient economy of the machine it may take longer to build up your endurance capacity to the level necessary to achieve a proper training effect . Most of the work is performed by the legs, so lactic acid build-up in these muscles and the resultant onset of fatigue is a real possibility. In swimming you use your whole body and even though it seems like more work, all your muscles are helping to pump the blood back to the heart and lungs where it is re-oxygenated. When cycling you can't circulate the blood fast enough into and out of your legs since this is where most of the demand for oxygen and glucose is. Consequently a competitive cyclist will use up to 10 per cent of his available energy in the musculature of the breathing apparatus; diaphragm, intercostals, abdominals, etc, in order to maintain as high a minute ventilation rate as possible – up to 200 litres per minute – to load the blood with oxygen which must find its way through a bottleneck (so to speak) to his legs.

Cycling obviously strengthens the muscles of the legs and buttocks as well as the heart and respiratory muscles. It is a good complementary sport to skating and both downhill and cross-country skiing. Since it is usually feasible to use cycling as a mode of transport, it is, along with walking, *the* sport for travel, touring and cross-country jaunts. Because of the adaptability to sightseeing, socializing or practical transport, cycling must be considered a prime sport for endurance and cardiovascular conditioning. As with other forms of endurance training, cycle for a minimum of 30 minutes three to six days a week in order to achieve a noticeable training effect. As you become fitter, remember to check your pulse to ensure that you are maintaining a work rate within your training sensitive zone (see page 105).

As a cyclist progresses towards more sophisticated riding skills and equipment, ability to maintain balance becomes more crucial. Weaving in and out of other cyclists, or for that matter, commuter traffic, requires visual acuity and an expanded spatial awareness. Looking over one's shoulder whilst maintaining direction requires an innate sense of balance. (Riding without using the handlebars is the product of balance and efficient posture.) Once these basic skills are acquired anyone can enjoy the training benefits of cycling.

At the competitive level, whether in road racing, criterium or pursuit racing, cycling becomes a game of strategy and tactics, demanding an intellectual involvement in planning your overall approach – when to stay with the pack, when to press your opponent, when to make a break.

At the recreational level cycling offers great opportunity for social interaction. Day trips, picnics or more extended tours all provide the occasion to be with friends away from the distractions of normal routines. The length of a cycling trip provides the right context for genuine relaxation as well. Remember, a 45-minute squash game is not enough to break chronic stress production patterns in your life, whereas an extended jaunt on a bicycle will do this and more. The connection with nature is a fundamental element of recreational riding. Many tourers describe this feeling and it seems to be a fundamental reason why this sport is so popular. The sense of unity that one experiences through the rhythm of the riding and the exposure to the open countryside rivals the joys described by the cross-country skiers surrounded by the white stillness of winter.

At a competitive level the dedication and self-discipline demanded by cycling is substantial. All cyclists, and road racers in particular, are known for their tremendous drive and self-mastery.

Injuries are not in themselves that common amongst recreational cyclists – it is far easier on the foot, knee and hip than running. Back problems are common but are usually due to improper form and can be overcome with adequate instruction. Heat strokes must be considered when riding in unusually hot weather and are best avoided by ensuring adequate drinking supplies and, in some cases, covering the head. On the other hand, colds usually result from extended exposure to inclement weather or when you are going through repeated changes between sweaty uphill slogs and gentle downhill coasts. But the major danger in cycling is the motorist. Collision while cycling is the single most common cause of injuries in all recreational sports. (In the USA in 1980 there were 537,100 hospitalizations from bicycling, 438,860 from baseball, and 425,300 for football). While a large percentage of these are in the 5–14 age group it still pays to take the necessary precautions to avoid injury.

Tennis

Tennis typifies contemporary sport. With its international venues, national competitions, glamorous millionaire champions and throngs of supporters, it has become a true 'megasport'. With so much focus on players' private lives, new young stars like Boris Becker and established favourites like Chris Lloyd, it is little wonder that tennis is such big news and big business.

Yet, it is a wonder to trace its origins back to the middle ages where it was first played by the monks in their monasteries, hitting the balls without racquets off the walls and sloping roofs of the cloisters. In fact, this game still exists almost intact and is played in special indoor courts under the name of 'real tennis'.

Tennis, originally 'jeu de paume', was played passionately by the French aristocracy throughout the fourteenth and fifteenth centuries and subsequently picked up by the other European courts. In fact the scoring of the game derives from the English aristocracy's addiction to sport and gambling. Each game was traditionally played for a crown – 60 pence. Thus the points scored were worth 15, 30, 45 (shortened to 40) and game (60 pence or a crown). It seems possible that the score of Love derives from the French *l'oeuf:* an egg, or zero.

Tennis has always been a social sport. While competition at any level is usually fierce, the tennis club provides for social ambience. And for most of us who play at the local public courts the contacts made with friends, arranging appointments, sharing a drink or a meal afterwards, all create a feeling of joining with others in a shared recreation.

Tennis helps maintain our sense of well being and physical training, but it is necessary to attain a certain degree of proficiency before you actually begin to see the physical benefits. Conditioning in tennis varies depending upon the kind of game you play. Serve and volley players will get very little aerobic conditioning out of their game but will develop some fast twitch muscle power as they put out repeated bursts of power and speed. If, however, you play a back-court game, and hit the ball hard and long over an extended period you may achieve a moderate amount of aerobic conditioning. But it will be limited. The average tennis point only lasts three seconds!

As tennis by itself does not really cultivate flexibility, stretching exercises, yoga classes, stretch classes are all a valuable complement. Good joint flexibility is particularly necessary in the upper body as the range of motion of the shoulder joint approaches 270 degrees in the service. Flexibility is also essential for scooping up low shots off the surface, rotating the torso to reach shots and in changing direction as rapidly as possible.

Depending upon your personal experience or 'school of thought', other racquet games either enhance your performance by training further hand-eye coordination, or may interfere with your tennis form by confusing your neuromuscular co-ordination in terms of the specific wrist, swing and body positioning components of your technique. We don't take a position in this particular controversy since it's your experience which counts.

Tennis, more than many sports, is dependent upon your ability to master and direct your control system. As such, it ranks high in terms of answering self-mastery and achievement aims. It takes a lot of practice to control the swing of your racquet, direct the ball across the net and intercept your opponent's shots. Anticipation is a key element in any competitive tennis player's mastery of the game. At the speed competitive tennis is played the eye cannot actually track the ball as it travels through its arc but rather picks it out at sequential points along its trajectory. The ability to anticipate the direction of the ball and where to place your racquet to meet this trajectory is a key factor in top level success. It is certainly apparent in the effortless game of John McEnroe, and Martina Navratilova's impeccable net game.

Many of the same basic motor skills and neuromuscular coordination which are a prerequisite for a successful alpine skier are also essential in tennis. There are only a limited number of strokes in tennis: forehand, backhand, forehand volley, backhand volley, service/smash, etc. They must be learned and if you are struggling with the neuromuscular and motor skills necessary to coordinate sound basic strokes and store them in your motor memory, then it is going to be extremely difficult to generalize these skills to all the variations of speed, distance, height and direction required to meet the ball from its multitude of trajectories and redirect it along the flight path of your choosing. It is important when learning to play tennis to have good instruction at the beginning so that you acquire the basic skills which will then have to be adapted to all the requirements of a well rounded game. Badly learned basics are very difficult to change at a later date. Resisting the temptation to play to win at an early stage in your tennis career is essential for acquiring good basic skills.

Tennis requires all-round coordination, quick reactions,

sharp visual acuity and good anticipation. You won't prevent heart attacks through playing tennis and you won't become Charles Atlas but you will achieve a sense of mastery over a game which requires good coordination, intelligent play and friendly interaction with your friends and partners.

Alpine Skiing

There are records of the practice of gliding over snow on wooden runners in cave drawings in Rodoy, Norway, which date from 2000 BC. It is the oldest form of travel on land, after walking, and quickly developed into a sophisticated mode of transport. By the sixteenth century it had been adopted by the military in Sweden. It began to be practised as a sport only in the 1850s, starting with slalom competitions in Scandinavia. Cross-country races were also common and in 1883 the Norwegian ski association was founded. However it was in Europe, in the Swiss, German and Austrian Alps that skiing really began to develop into the popular sport it is today.

The advance in alpine skiing was due in part to the development of sophisticated skis by Matthias Zdarsky, an Austrian army officer, which enabled greater manoeuverability over the more inconsistent terrain of the Alps, and in part to the great concentration in Europe of the rich and leisured. By 1900 the functional Scandinavian system of winter travel had been transformed into an exciting sport for those with the time, money and audacity. In 1928 the first winter Olympics were held in St Moritz, with first one nation then another dominating the skiing scene. Now, what was formerly only a rich man's sport has opened its doors to people from all walks of life.

Downhill skiing is an anaerobic sport since, unless you are an expert skier, the demand placed on the body is not consistent enough, nor is your pulse sustained at the training level for a long enough period of time to provide aerobic conditioning. At the elementary level runs are too short, or the skier falls. Yet skiing may make exceptional demands upon the beginner and it is common to have to stop from being out of breath, experiencing burning thighs or shaky legs from this unfamiliar effort. Very important at every level of skiing is a high anaerobic threshold and the ability to 'blow off' CO_2, which rids the muscles of lactic acid build-up. Both these abilities are enhanced through aerobic training so even though skiing is essentially anaerobic it is beneficial to undertake some form of aerobic conditioning prior to a skiing trip as this will increase your recovery rate and enhance the satisfaction you derive from skiing.

Off-season training could involve cycling since this trains many of the same muscles used in skiing: quadriceps in the thighs, gluteus in the buttocks and the oblique and rectus muscles of the abdomen. The aerobic training from cycling makes you fitter and the transition to the slope more effortless. Risk of injury is also reduced by off-season training, circuit training, soccer, dance, tae kwon do or any movement form which gives you intense bursts of activity while also increasing your aerobic capacity. This is especially relevant to beginners since so often those precious two weeks are spent suffering from grievously aching legs and knees which can mean spending more time falling than skiing.

One of the key requirements for downhill skiing is visual acuity. Skiing requires a high degree of anticipation; picking one's way through obstacles, looking ahead, choosing a line through a field of moguls, adjusting to changing weather and snow conditions. Balance and proprioceptive feedback are essential components of skiing ability. Maintaining oneself erect through a whole range of manoeuvres, few of which bear any relation to daily movement, and many of which run counter to our balancing techniques when on the flat, all require the ability to see and assess quickly the best course and to feel what messages the piste is giving you through your feet, ankles, knees and the balancing devices in your inner ear. This last receptor alerts the skier whenever his balance is thrown off; your limb receptors allow you to know where your arms and legs are without looking so you can position yourself properly for a turn; proprioceptors in ankles and feet help determine how much ski edge is necessary, feel the chattering of the skis as they hit an icy patch, and where the knees are – forward or backwards, left or right of the midline; receptors of the feet give information as to how far forward or backward your whole body is on your skis, and your lateral movements.

This information feedback must be accompanied by substantial motor abilities. Timing, balance, agility, coordination, are essential to your skiing ability. When the Austrians set themselves the task, in the 1960s, of overtaking the French, they established a testing programme in which ten-year olds were given 32 different motor ability tests designed to select for ski training the children with the highest possible amount of motor coordination and ability.

Downhill skiing certainly does require a higher degree of motor ability and coordination than most other sports and to progress beyond a standard level requires the ability to learn new skills and interrupt old patterns. The level of skill required in skiing involves the essential overriding of a number of re-flexive or deep-seated patterns of response. The proliferation of ski schools and alternative coaching methods, such as Inner Skiing, in comparison to other sports, points to the fact that skiing is difficult to learn and requires knowledgeable coaching. Skiing requires a good kinaesthetic sense: to be able not only to visualize, but also to feel your position in space and how you should organize your movements; as well as a more than average amount of genetic material to work with in the form of sensory feedback, motor ability and learning skills.

Injuries, particularly traumatic ones, have declined over the last ten to fifteen years, partly as a result of the publicity they got and the subsequent increase in thorough and effective teaching. In addition, scientifically designed boots and more sophisticated release mechanisms on the bindings have decreased the injury risk. Injuries are now largely caused by the skier: lack of training and conditioning; inadequate warming up; too much glüwein at lunch; adventurous experimentation on the last day of the holiday when fatigue has built up. Skiing is a potentially dangerous sport, fast and complex. Full attention to the risks involved, concentration on the slopes and sensible preparation in lessons and warming up will greatly lessen the risks and make sure you enjoy your skiing rather than just survive it.

Cross-Country Skiing

Cross-country skiing has much the same pedigree as Alpine skiing, but the fact that they are classified as two entirely different sports gives a clue to the fundamental difference between the fast, athletic, bursts of speed down a precipitous mountainside and the methodical long distance touring of the cross-country skier. While Alpine skiing is a sport which relies heavily on power and fast twitch muscle fibres, with very high demands upon skill and anticipation, cross-country skiing is, in many ways, the preeminent cardiovascular and endurance sport.

Bill Koch, the 1983 World Cup champion, and everyone's model of the ideal cross-country skier, has developed both the cardiovascular fitness and massive lung capacity necessary in cross-country skiing and has brought with it superb motor skills and coordination which has allowed him to turn the downhill portions of his run into displays of power and skill, achieving speeds of 60 miles an hour and more, often rivalling the speed of Alpine skiers. Just to keep up with demands of the high tech skis and the increasingly challenging courses, cross-country skiers require motor abilities approaching those of a top downhill skier and the endurance capacities of a top marathon runner.

As a conditioning and training sport, many people place cross-country skiing at the top of their list as an all round form of exercise. Not only does it cultivate cardiovascular fitness and endurance capabilities, but it also uses most of the muscles of the body. In addition it requires good overall coordination and both gross motor control and multi-limb coordination. Cross-country skiing is an almost entirely aerobic exercise. Sven-Ake Lundbäck, the Swedish Olympic Gold medal winner in cross-country skiing, has the highest oxygen consumption capacity ever measured: 94 mm per kilo. Since oxygen consumption is a good way of measuring the body's capacity to sustain constant effort, it reflects other factors like heart size, lung capacity, and particularly the actual ability of the muscle cells to utilize a large quantity of oxygen. And since oxygen utilization is usually much greater in slow twitch fibres than fast twitch fibres, it is not too surprising that someone with Lundbäck's ability to utilize oxygen would be able to maintain a high work rate and still function aerobically.

Lung capacity in athletes seems to be higher amongst cross-country skiers than any other sport, marathon running and swimming included. This is partially due to the fact that a large boned and fairly mesomorphic individual is ideally suited to cross-country skiing, so many top cross-country skiers are genetically inclined towards large lung capacities. But that aside, more body muscles are used than in any other sport, even more than swimming. As well as the obvious use of calves, thighs, arms and shoulder muscles, the muscles of the buttocks, chest, abdomen, lower back and upper back are all used, hence the very high demand for oxygen to fuel all of the muscles over the length of the course. This high utilization of energy is reflected in the tremendous generation of body heat. During the pre-Olympic games at Lake Placid in 1979 when temperatures were as low as -22F, skiers still wore relatively little clothing and one skier, Juha Mieto, wore only a single skintight suit and no gloves at all!

At the beginner's level anyone can put on a pair of cross-country skis and travel across a snowy landscape. It is easy, it is fun and it is definitely good exercise. In fact, it is very demanding and first time skiers will find their progress often exhausting. Developing a good cross-country skiing technique is not that easy – again the peculiar scissoring glide and kick technique combined with conscious use of the arms in poling is unfamiliar and will take a good while to develop. Cross-country skiing, like running and swimming, can be enjoyed at any level of skill but is quite demanding and arduous until your cardiovascular fitness has been developed to the point where you can sustain the effort below the anaerobic threshold for the particular sport. In the case of cross-country skiing this seems to be moderately higher than the other aerobic sports.

There is no particular sport which is an ideal complement to cross-country skiing in the off season. Cycling involves similar leg movements and also helps the individual deal with the hills and slopes in a way similar to the demands of cross-country skiing. Running will help build leg resistance but uses different ratios of leg muscles. Some cross-country skiers train in the summer by running up and down hills, thus mirroring the general use of the muscles more and also the up and down demand upon the cardiovascular system. Swimming and rowing don't use the same muscle patterns as in cross-country skiing, though they do build up the muscles of the arms and back.

In terms of muscle fibre, even though cross-country skiing is preeminently an endurance sport, it does require some mixture of fast twitch fibres with slow twitch fibres. The poling movement in the arms and shoulders is usually very fast and explosive, sometimes exceeding more than 400 degress of rotation per second.

Cross-country skiing produces relatively few injuries and those few are due to over-use. It is not as tough on knees and ankles as running or bicycling, and the risks of traumatic injuries are much less than in Alpine skiing. Sprains and twists, not the least in the thumb, do occur but the main concern is catching cold. Because you generate so much heat it is important to wear clothing in layers which can be peeled off as you warm up. Sweating from over heating combined with sudden drops in temperature can result in frost-bite or hypothermia, as the sweat freezes against your skin. Like cycling, plenty of fluids should be drunk, but steer clear of alcoholic beverages as these dilate the blood vessels near your skin, resulting in abrupt heat loss.

If you have any kind of heart disease, it is best to consult a doctor about cross-country skiing since it places such high demands upon your heart.

Soccer

Soccer is an international sport and the most widely played of all team games. It is a passionate, thrilling and demanding game, the source of tremendous national pride and celebration and a language which can bridge ethnic and national chasms. It has its antecedents in the earliest history of games.

Variations of football itself first began to appear throughout Europe under a variety of different names during the middle ages. As the names varied so did the rules. Sometimes whole villages played, as with the annual Shrove Tuesday match played in the thirteenth century between the parishes of St Peter's and All Saints in Derby. The pitch was the three miles that separated the waterwheel at All Saints and the town gate of St Peter's! Kicking, running, pushing, biting and tackling . . . anything went. More than one old score was settled during the day-long competition.

By the nineteenth century football was played all over the world. In England it was the game of public schoolboys, though rules differed from school to school. By the 1850s the game had settled into two primarily different styles: the field game which resembled contemporary soccer and the Rugby form with its running, passing and scrums. In 1863 the Football Association was formed, setting down a number of rules including no running with the ball or throwing or passing. Handling was eliminated in 1871. There were then fifty clubs in the Football Association – by 1900 there were over ten thousand! A separate association had been formed to organize Rugby-style football, and football itself became known as soccer, a derivation from the abbreviation of Association to Assoc. to soccer.

European nations followed suit and in 1893 an international football association was founded. South America in turn caught the bug and in fact the first World Cup competition was held in Uruguay in 1930. The working class involvement in football became more prominent in Britain as the Midlands and the Northern counties began to dominate the Football Association. It was twenty years after the founding of the Football Association that the Blackburn Olympics (which included three weavers, a picture framer, an iron foundry worker, a spinner and a dental assistant) beat the Old Etonians in 1883.

After the Depression, football emerged as a powerful, highly paid sport with international appeal and its own World Cup competition outside the Olympics. More than 200,000 filled the Maracana Stadium in Rio de Janeiro for the 1950 World Cup Final. In addition television has invaded the pitch. In 1972 800 million people watched the televised World Cup final in Mexico City. To this day there is no single team sport which approaches soccer in its international appeal.

Soccer is a good cardiovascular conditioner but the overall energy requirements during a game are approximately 30 per cent aerobic and 70 per cent anaerobic. You need to be able to maintain a high work rate running up and down the pitch but the start and stop nature of the game gives the player a chance to rest and catch his breath, thus lowering the heart rate below the training level which produces an aerobic conditioning effect. At any given time in the match you might be required to make a long offensive run and then, finding your side dispossessed, have to dash back the length of the field in order to make a vital defensive run. This places strong demands on your phosphagen and lactic acid systems and hence requires good anaerobic energy production.

As might be expected, most good soccer players have a relatively even mixture of fast twitch and slow twitch muscle fibres in order to be able to run the length of the field repeatedly and also to deliver suddenly a powerful kick to the ball. Most of this muscular development takes place in the lower body: hamstrings, gastrocnemius, quadraceps, gluteus muscles and the hip adductors and abductors are all used regularly.

Flexibility is an important factor. Only recently have professional players paid more than lip service to stretching. But the sustained use of the muscles of the lower body suggests that attention should be paid to stretching during the warming up period and at the end of a match as well. Football is a game of sudden movements, abrupt stops, changes in direction, leaps over an intended tackle and other such acrobatics. Because of this, flexibility exercises should involve a fair degree of range of movement. Yoga is valuable, but movement systems like t'ai chi, Feldenkrais and even dance training will suit football players better. Any intensive stretching training should be accompanied by some form of muscle strengthening around the joints as well.

Soccer requires a good deal of neuromuscular coordination to perform well and yet individuals with minimal skills can still participate. Most of us can run, jump, dodge and kick. These are the motor programmes basic to soccer which is one reason why it is such a popular sport. However the ball handling skills required at higher levels of performance allow the individual with innate ability to excel in controlling the ball, dribbling, volleying, regulating the force and direction of a kick, curling the ball and so on.

Another reason why soccer is so popular is because it allows individuals with different skills and personalities to play in different positions. Defensive, midfield and offensive players are three different creatures altogether. Football allows for varying heights and sizes. It is one sport where the small person can often have an advantage, with his low centre of gravity, close contact with the ground and ease of ability to change directions.

In terms of injuries, there are always a regular number of problems in football. If you play recreational football on the occasional weekend without any regular running, stretching or strengthening exercise, then you are opening the door to injury. As you get older, putting on additional weight without additional training, you increase the possibility of a serious ankle, knee or groin injury. If you don't play football enough to stay in shape then practise some other discipline like a martial art, squash or disco dancing (a wonderful conditioning system). Exercise which involves regular twisting and turning as football does will reduce the risk of injury during a match.

Football offers the opportunity of experiencing that thrill unique to team sports in which a long-practised tactic suddenly comes off and you feel that not only you yourself but you as a member of that greater whole, the team, have achieved a special goal. Moments like these are often reward enough to ensure a continued commitment to the sport by individuals at all levels all over the world.

Volleyball

In spite of its widespread popularity, volleyball is a relatively new sport. It was literally invented in 1895 in Holyoke, Massachusetts by William G. Morgan, the local YMCA director. He wanted to create a game which middle aged men could play instead of basketball which they found too demanding. The game took off beyond anyone's expectations and by the 1900's was already being played in Canada, the Philippines, and South America; by WW1 it was being played all over Europe. The International Volleyball Federation (LVBF) was established in 1947 to coordinate the sport and organize competitions worldwide. The Russians soon emerged as world leaders but it was really the 1964 Olympics which thrust volleyball into the limelight. In those games the Japanese women's teams emerged from nowhere to capture the Gold medal in an amazing exhibition of coordination, and acrobatics. They also won the hearts of the world audience with their dedication, their inspired team spirit and their profound emotional commitment to their sport.

Volleyball is a truly popular international team sport, more widely played, after soccer, than any other team sport. It appeals equally to men and women, and everyone seems to be able to bat a volleyball over the net in the pick-up games which can be seen in any park or on any beach. But this is not volleyball as it is played competitively and anyone who is interested in volleyball as a sport will soon progress beyond the untutored free-for-all games you sometimes see.

At moderate levels of skill the sport is primarily anaerobic. Points last as long as a badminton point might last, usually longer than a tennis point. As each point is won, there is a stop, positions may be changed, service may be passed over to the team who wins the point. But at a top competitive level, the sport produces a fair degree of aerobic conditioning – points last longer, higher demands are made on the cardiovascular system, players are moving more about the court preparing for the next attack or organizing their own attack.

There are particularly strong demands upon the lower body in volleyball: you are constantly jumping to perform a spike, diving to reach a ball, squatting under a volley and generally running, leaping and propelling yourself about the court. If you are an attacker and perform a lot of spikes, then you will also develop upper body strength, and since spiking with either hand is encouraged, development will take place on both sides of the body. Since the pace of the whole game requires rapid and coordinated movement, volleyball is particularly good for cultivating neuromuscular skills and coordination. Anticipation is vital, more so, if possible, than tennis, as the court is so small and it is very easy to fake attacking shots. Hand–eye coordination is essential as well.

In addition to ball-handling skills (a slight misnomer, since except during service you are not actually allowed to 'hold' the ball), there are a large range of movement and positioning skills required for court coverage and tactics. There are also dives, rolls and lunges used to reach balls which do not come directly to you, so although volleyball in itself does not cultivate flexibility, it is good to practise flexibility training particularly for the lower body so that you can play the game energetically and to the full without the risk of pulling muscles. The main injuries seem to be jammed or sprained fingers and occasional sprained ankles but generally volleyball does not produce a lot of injuries. It is one of the few team sports (cricket is another) which is entirely free of body contact. Opponents are on the other side of the net and there are no injuries from clashes between opposing forces.

Because volleyball does not have the pedigree of cricket or soccer, it is inviting to everyone and anyone. It is a friendly and social game with a lot of goodwill amongst all of the players. Because of the size of the court, and the number of players, everyone participates and during a game there is ample opportunity to make contact with the ball. Increasingly volleyball is being played at high standards but most clubs will have A and B teams and, of course, men's and women's teams. There are clubs everywhere, in most colleges and universities, at most YMCAs and YWCAs. In addition there are a wide number of ethnic clubs. Most volleyball players feel that it provides the kind of physical and social atmosphere which is serious and yet more relaxed than for example, weekly squash games. Its widespread availability and the pleasure of accomplishment which accompanies regular practice makes volleyball a prime candidate for anyone interested in participation in a team sport.

Body Conditioning Methods

The whole notion of keeping fit has origins which predate the current surge of fitness training by thousands of years. The ancient Greeks, for instance, espoused physical well being as a core element of their culture, social life and martial pride. The realism of their sculpture directly reflects the value placed on physical beauty, and some of the basic principles of body proportion established as the ideal by the Greeks still very much influence our criteria for physical beauty and alignment today. The city state of Sparta enforced a widespread system of rigorously disciplined physical training and in Rome the notion of physical fitness was also associated with military discipline and prowess.

During the Renaissance fitnss and the body beautiful enjoyed an upsurge. Long before this monks had played games as part of a regime of health maintenance in their monasteries. And it is worth noting that the Eastern martial arts derive from the fitness regimes of Buddhist and Taoist monks as well. But as an organized system of physical training nowhere has 'fitness' as a concept been more systematically promulgated in the past than in Europe at the end of the 18th century. And its military character can be clearly seen in its development in the Prussian military tradition.

With the rise of Napoleon on the Continent, a German, Johann Friedrich GutsMuth, wrote his seminal work *Gymnastics for Youth* (1793). GutsMuth's guidelines were duplicated by Franz Nachtegall in Copenhagen and extended through a student of his, Per Henrik Ling in Sweden. The Danish Government appointed Nachtegall to train army officers in defence against Napoleon, and Ling was made director of the Royal Central Institute of Gymnastics in Stockholm. Gymnastics, as practised at the Institute, involved running, jumping, climbing, vaulting, indoors or outdoors, in a systematic way designed to increase levels of strength and fitness. But perhaps best known of the gymnasts during this period was another German, Friedrich Ludwig Jahn 'the father of German gymnastics'. His nationalistic pride smarting from the Prussian defeat by France, Jahn published his book *The German Way of Life* in 1810 and as part of his proposals to re-invigorate the German spirit, mind and body, set up playgrounds, or Turnplatzen, for children outside Berlin where they could practise and train in his form of gymnastics. The Prussian army employed his methods and his Turner (gymnastic) Society began to thrive around the country.

With the regularizing of sports which took place in the latter half of the nineteenth century, and their rise in popularity, an increased emphasis was placed on physical training and its study in the centres of higher education. By the beginning of the twentieth century a number of universities had established colleges of physical education. Sciences like physiology and anatomy were becoming respectable and more esoteric disciplines such as exercise physiology, biomechanics and kinesiology were being formulated. Not only was it respectable to play sport and train, it was also now perfectly acceptable to study the human being as a functioning organism that moved, exercised and excelled in physical performance.

With this new development of the study of human performance came the growth of movement systems with an emphasis on the therapeutic and health aspects rather than physical prowess solely for militaristic purposes. Europe was once again particularly fertile ground, with pioneers such as Laban and Dalcroze significantly changing concepts of physical fitness (for greater discussion of their work see Movement Awareness Techniques, pages 262–283). Movement educators tended to come from the world of dance or therapy rather than sport, and the combination of aesthetics with science influenced the character of gymnastics and physical training in Britain and Europe, moving from regimentation to more romantic notions of fitness, well being, the body beautiful and physical supremacy. Tragically this culminated in the final gross distortion of Hitler's Aryan Ideal. Once again physical fitness was being used to service national pride, and the inevitable result was that after the war in Europe fitness once more fell out of fashion.

In Britain, meanwhile, three individual women founded movements with the aim of improving the health of the nation, (but particularly that of women), which grew and developed during the 1930s, 40s and 50s.

Margaret Morris, a dancer, founded the Margaret Morris Movement in the early years of this century, combining elements from yoga, from dance (an artistic approach emphasizing colour and free-flowing movement), and later, from physiotherapy. MMM still flourishes with nearly half a million attendances at classes in Great Britain, and in international branches in Canada, Europe and Japan.

The Women's League of Health and Beauty was founded in 1930 by Mary Bagot Stack. The aim, as she puts it in her own account of her 'mission', was to cultivate 'racial health' plus the 'sparkle that most women love'. The League certainly carried the flavour of the period, with vigorous gymnastic exercises — the 'Bagot Stack System' – performed by robust young women during their morning routine and at mass rallies and displays. A woman with a vision and skilled at public relations, Mrs Bagot Stack established a nationwide network of classes and teaching centres fired by her belief that health and beauty would help furnish peace after the devastation of the First World War. Her naive beliefs seem today uncannily close to Jahn's regeneration of national pride and to the cultivation of health, youth and vigour during the inter-war years in Germany. She died in 1935, but in 1937 her daughter, who succeeded her in heading the League, was invited (as was Margaret Morris) to serve on the newly formed National Fitness Council for England and Wales. The League is now a worldwide organization with centres in Britain, Europe, South Africa, New Zealand and Canada.

The Keep Fit Association is perhaps the best known of the three movements largely because they have consistently updated their public image and kept to the forefront of sports and physical education politics. Founded by Norah Reed, a physical education organizer, in the 1930s, the movement aimed to encourage exercise participation as well as a better understanding of the general principles of movement. Unlike the other two organizations the KFA has remained a national body with regional offices throughout the country.

Through the influence of organizations such as these, gymnastic style classes attracted an overwhelmingly female clientele. Men, on the other hand, were pursuing the avenues opened up to them through sport. With the war over and finished, the last thing any man wanted to be reminded of was military training. Body conditioning techniques for men followed the footsteps of sport, and physical training became recreational. Competition took the form of games, not life and death confrontations. But for the vast majority of men over 25, games became something you played at school or university; or at the outside they would occasionally kick a ball around on a Sunday afternoon. And with the arrival of television in the 1950s, sport as a passive pastime blossomed. Two factors interrupted this gradual slide into lethargy. The first was the President's Council of Physical Fitness instituted by the American President, John F. Kennedy, in the early 1960s. The second was the development of the science of epidemiology (the study of disease trends in population groups). By the 1960s the link between the deterioration of our health due to our increasingly sedentary lifestyle and the role of exercise in maintaining it was made with ever greater insistence. Gradually organized exercise on a regular basis with an emphasis on health maintenance – as opposed to sports training or sport for recreation – began to enjoy a popular revival.

This new surge of activity came not from Europe but from the United States and one of its principal exponents and popularizers was Dr Kenneth Cooper. Again the background is a military one: Cooper was a lieutenant colonel in the medical corps of the US Air Force, and the development of his Aerobics Points system was founded on research conducted over many years with Air Force personnel. Eventually his system was to replace the routines of calisthenics, gymnastics and circuit training, as the official keep fit programme of the American military.

Cooper's books, the first published in 1968, made available to the general public the information and techniques which enabled them to organize their own keep fit programmes along rational but personal lines. This moved keep fit away from the tedium of repetitive exercises and the authoritarian or the romantic image. Now each individual could test his or her present fitness level, choose among a number of 'aerobic' activities and work out a personal schedule of exercise according to how many points he or she needed to attain. It is a complex game, finding your way around Cooper's charts, but one that has appealed to millions.

With this renewed awareness of the body, muscles were becoming fashionable. Weight training techniques and equipment became more scientific and methodical. Sports people who for years had shied away from weights precisely because of the 'bodybuilding' image associated with them, watched top athletes being churned out of the Eastern Bloc countries during the 1950s. It was their extensive, scientifically monitored weight training regimes which contributed to their success. With the 'me' generation of the 60s came an increased open admiration for physical beauty and perfection. Don't-let-them-kick-sand-in-your-face Charles Atlas was replaced by the Arnold Schwarzenegger phenomenon and film stars like Sylvester Stallone. The Weider brothers built a financial empire around the marketing of body-building equipment and magazines. What had formerly been an impulse from a teenager to build up his biceps so that he could carry a pack of cigarettes in the rolled up sleeve of his T-shirt became a mainstream and upmarket fascination with muscle.

While bodybuilding and weight training muscled into the male fitness scene, the perennial female desire to be thin, risen to manic levels in the 60s and 70s, joined with the willpower and independence emphasized by the growing women's movement. Fashion, too, jumped into the scene, emphasizing these elements and capturing a huge female market, first in leotards, leg warmers and jogging shoes (as well as expanding its male market in sports and fitness equipment and gear), then secondly in the sports and leisure wear sector for both sexes. All of these social elements fuelled the rise of fitness as a way of life.

Film stars began to reflect this massive social trend and offer confessions of their personal fitness regimes. Jane Fonda was one of the first to capture a truly mass following injecting a huge shot of Hollywood glamour into keeping fit with her *Workout* book, published in 1981. Her entry on the scene marked a new fanaticism affecting primarily women but also men. Exercise classes gave way in conversation to 'the workout'. Keeping fit was now a matter of sweat, pant and the notorious 'burn'. The female image became honed, muscled, harder and more determined – the superwoman cult. Leotards were cut higher on the thigh revealing more of the flesh every woman was exhorted to get rid of. Soon some form of strenuous exercise was seen as a prerequisite of the glamorous image for star and fashionable woman alike. The fitness boom has sparked a re-examination of roles by both women and men. Men started to go to exercise or 'aerobics' classes. But perhaps more revolutionary, women have invaded the gymnasium. Where once a woman might have been looked at askance if she admitted to attending exercise classes to maintain her figure it was now a social must to belong to a gym, go running, work out, swim or play some sport.

The sporty, healthy, relaxed image is, it seems, here to stay in the pantheon of fashionable 'looks'. Superficial as it may at first appear, this shift has had a profound effect on women's and men's lives. It is now perfectly acceptable for women to appear attractive in loose, comfortable clothing made from sports fabrics, and to wear flat, casual shoes. Men can wear jogging outfits to a wide variety of social occasions, even, sometimes, to work. Comfort has become a hallmark of style. These details of how we see and present ourselves in the world have made a significant difference to the ease and quality of daily life. In the case of women the option to adopt a style that reflects being active and strong rather than a passive and pretty object, in high heels and tight skirts, for instance, has helped broaden women's images of themselves and their roles in society.

With the capitalization of the business and fashion worlds on this mass bid from individuals for a fitter, healthier life, the body conditioning scene moved swiftly into a phase of hype and counter-hype. Classes mushroomed too rapidly for anyone to be really aware of what was happening. With the lack of supervisory bodies in Britain, and the lure of fast money and public demand, people with the minimum of training started teaching exercise classes – usually dubbed 'aerobics'. The emphasis shifted from Cooper's pulse checks and graded exercise to glamour and speed, to the imitation of a style rather than the teaching of a tried and tested technique. The more established forms of keep fit were drowned out in this California-inspired blast. If the music was loud, enthusiasm and fun high, if the students sweated profusely and ached after class, this was seen to be enough.

This state of affairs inevitably led to a huge increase in injuries both among students and their inexperienced teachers.

While physiotherapists reaped the benefits, many voices in the sports and exercise field decried the lack of standards, safety measures and a governing body to monitor and stop the 'cowboys'.

In Britain three bodies were set up under the aegis of the Exercise Federation: The Central Affiliation of Professional Exercise Teachers (CAPET), the Independent Dance Exercise and Aerobics Society (IDEAS) and the Aerobic Fitness Teachers Association (AFTA). There was fierce discussion and disagreement among these organizations, but in 1985 CAPET and IDEAS amalgamated to become ASSET and it is to be hoped that the consequent strengthening of their power will enable them soon to fulfil their purpose: to prescribe national safety guidelines, procedural format and the setting up and monitoring of much-needed teacher training courses in exercise classes.

In this section we outline some of the major forms of exercise which have body conditioning as their sole aim. Some have been established for years, others are new developments. There are hundreds of different classes, systems, training regimes and many different weight training methods and machines to choose from. While the individual style of a class or technique will reflect the training, bias and personality of the teacher, most will be a version of the following principal methods. We do not offer these as the only ones worthy of pursuit, but rather as guidelines. They will help you pinpoint the factors that should concern you when choosing a training regime amongst the classes and equipment available to you.

Keep Fit

Keep fit has been one of the best known exercise forms in terms of organized classes in Britain since the 1930s, when the keep fit movement was started by Norah Reed in the Sunderland area of the north of England, with the aim of promoting a positive attitude to health through physical fitness for all social classes. Norah Reed stressed in her manual that there should be a real mix of women attending keep fit classes and even introduced a uniform of tunic and matching knickers to bridge the gap between the poor and the better off. She recognized the need for crêche facilities and for women to meet socially, free of household duties for an evening. This was very much in the spirit of the pioneering health projects of the period before the Second World War when the social aspects of health were starting to be recognized and acted upon. Health for all became a matter of political conscience and initiative, health centres were set up, and publicity campaigns and a great variety of projects were put into practice to raise public consciousness of their own health and well being.

While the two other widespread exercise networks for women at this time, the Women's League for Health and Beauty and the Margaret Morris Movement, have their roots in visions of peace and enhanced femininity and beauty through flowing exercise and dance routines, Norah Reed's inspiration came from the gymnastics classes she saw on visits to Denmark and Sweden. Keep Fit had from the start a hale and hearty, 'northern' feel to it. It was also based on the movement principles devised by Rudolph Laban who pioneered a form of movement notation much used by dancers and those interested in the psychological aspects of movement. Laban was also involved with improving the fitness of factory workers and teaching physical education in schools.

After the Second World War the Keep Fit movement grew, teachers were trained and classes sprang up all over the country. In 1956 a national association was set up, as a voluntary body, grant aided by the Sports Council. This sets it apart from the aerobics, body conditioning and other fitness classes which have come on the scene since. As such it is the official voice for the promotion and teaching of keep fit in Britain and its qualifications are recognized by education authorities.

A keep fit teacher is taught body mechanics and function, Laban's analysis of movement, the use of music in exercise teaching, and first aid. The style of classes reflects this thorough two year training. Classes are disciplined and organized, although the pace of them will be geared to the level and needs of participants. The type of exercises are modified gymnastics: jumping jacks, stretches, bends, lunges and windmills done to music (rather than to orders from the gym mistress). There are no aerobic style routines and the Association is keen to avoid the word, given the controversies that surround the teaching of aerobic workouts. None the less they have clearly been influenced by research done into the benefits of aerobic exercise and this is reflected in the present division of their classes into a warm-up period of slow movements followed by a faster routine and ending with a slower cool down. The exact proportion and composition of these three sections will depend on the individual teacher. In recent years keep fit teachers have added the use of props to their classes to give variety to an essentially gym style of exercise. Rather than simply repeating turns, jumps and lunges, students now do exercises with hoops, balls, clubs, skipping ropes and ribbons. Many of the classes are geared to preparation for local demonstrations or for the annual London event. The style is one of smooth, synchronised movement with a gymnastic rather than dance or acrobatic flavour. Classes last about an hour and teachers will coach their students rather than teach by imitation. Teachers are encouraged to develop their own style so it will depend on the initiative, imagination and personality of the individual teacher as to how lively or old-fashioned a keep fit class may be. The Association puts no limit on the number of participants, which may be as many as 50 or 60, depending on the size of the venue.

During the 1960s Keep Fit lost popularity due to its rather stuffy image and, with the influx of more free-form and glamorous techniques from Europe and the United States, there is as yet no sign of a mass popular revival. But the KFA is still a powerful body, recognized by the Sports Council, with a big say in who gets funding or research grants. It also runs a comprehensive and sound part-time training course. Classes are still widespread throughout Britain, but are nowadays more than likely to be called by names such as Fitness to Music. Even when not signalled as Keep Fit, the techniques and coaching methods are widely used by the teachers trained by the Association, and since these are so well established and so thorough KFA credentials are worth noting when exploring exercise options.

Body Conditioning

All methods of body conditioning have behind them the same

basic goals: to promote flexibility and suppleness, and in some cases strength, of the muscles and joints, through stretching and isotonic exercises. Some body conditioning teachers have incorporated faster moving exercises to promote cardiovascular fitness into their programme. But in general you can expect to find exercises that derive from one or several of the following: yoga, dance warm-ups and toning exercises, gymnastics, calisthenics and acrobatics and various therapeutic techniques. You may not recognize them as such for every teacher will combine, adapt, modify and develop these exercises according to her own style and the needs and demands of the class.

Body conditioning classes are often done to music but tend to be slow and deliberate rather than fluid, bouncy or performance orientated. Every part of the body is exercised in isolation and a class will include exercises for toning, for flexibility, for suppleness and for strength. There should be a balance between standing work, floor work and, in some cases, barre work. Exercises are done on the spot rather than moving through space. Many teachers will use the format of setting eight repetitions for every movement; some, following the example of yoga, require their students to hold one position for a prolonged period of time; some believe in the value of the dynamic stretching of muscles, others in static stretching (see Flexibility pages 111–119). Most emphasize the importance of posture (something to look for when choosing a class). A good teacher should put some emphasis on relaxing tension, particularly in the upper body, perhaps incorporating a relaxation session at the end of the class.

Lotte Berk is a renowned figure in the body conditioning world. Born in 1931 she is considered one of the *grandes dames* of fitness exercise, since there was a period when hers was the only exercise classes available in London which offered a sophisticated and hard-working alternative to the Keep Fit Association or the Margaret Morris Movement.

Lotte Berk's early career was in modern ballet, first as a star in the Germany of the twenties, and then, after fleeing Nazi persecution, on the stages of England, from Covent Garden, and the Glyndebourne and Edinburgh festivals, to popular musicals and the night clubs of London. Her life centred on the glittering Bohemia of England's avant garde art world of the

1930s, and she mixed with the stars of theatre, dance, music and painting. She brings this background to her style of teaching: a mix of rigorous dance and orthopaedic exercises (which she studied later after damaging her spine in an accident).

Her 45-minute classes are characterized by their toughness. Long before Jane Fonda made her mark, her students would emerge from their first lesson with Lotte Berk, their legs like jelly. The pace is continuous, and punctuated, if taught by Lotte herself, with her caustic, cheeky comments, thus setting the style – a kind of challenging approach – for the many teachers she has trained.

The reason for the jelly legs at the end of even several sessions of Lotte Berk is the foundation of her exercises on basic ballet training and positions: a larger part of her classes than is usual in body conditioning is devoted to strengthening the legs. Calves, thighs, inner and outer, quads and buttocks are all worked to burning point. Emphasis throughout is put on building strength more than on flexibility, suppleness or awareness.

Over the years Lotte Berk has trained many teachers and her method has spread, although there is still a certain exclusivity to her classes. For those wanting a really strenuous body conditioning method based on sound techniques of modern ballet (if perhaps over-exacting for the lay person), then Lotte Berk is one choice. She predates Jane Fonda by at least a decade, but the rigorous style and ballet basis are very similar. Make sure that you start with a beginners' class if one is available, and if not, don't push yourself as hard as the teacher may urge. There is absolutely no virtue in straining a muscle to its maximum and beyond. Take it slowly and build up your strength gradually.

A very different style of working altogether is the method evolved by Barbara Dale. **Bodywork** is a method of body conditioning based on the work of the American movement specialist, Bess Mensendieck. Barbara Dale has been running a training course for teachers of exercise for some time so her methods have become widespread, her influence also extending through her long involvement with the world of movement and dance in an advisory, teaching and, latterly, administrative capacity as one of the founder members of CAPET (see page 193). Her way of working is typical of those who take a slower, quasi-therapeutic approach to exercise.

The emphasis in Bodywork is on body awareness as well as on conditioning every part of the body to function at its best. Barbara Dale's training was in ballet, Alexander Technique, then the Martha Graham method of contemporary dance and the movement analysis of Rudolph Laban. It was her encounter with the Mensendieck Method that began the development of a thorough, safe and non-violent keep fit method for the lay person.

Barbara Dale learnt and then taught the method and gradually adapted and enriched it with elements from her other training. She was one of the first exercise teachers to put especial emphasis on incorporating a proper period of relaxation at the end of her classes. This came out of her studies with the relaxation expert Laura Mitchell. Likewise one of Barbara's principal teachers took time off to study the renowned movement awareness teacher in Paris, Thérèse Bertherat. Many of her methods – such as for example, the use of small, hard balls held between floor and wall and parts of the body to increase subtle awareness – are now incorporated into some of the classes.

The basic Bodywork class is 75 minutes long. All classes, beginners, intermediate or advanced begin with warm-up exercises, starting with the head, neck and shoulders. Care is taken to give precise instructions and classes are kept small so that the teacher can see exactly what each student is doing. Continuity is emphasized so students pay for a term's classes in advance. They are encouraged to start with the basic class and progress from there.

The intermediate and advanced classes now incorporate a session of aerobic movement — continuous jumps, running on the spot, kicks, jumping jacks, and simple bouncy dance steps – for 15–20 minutes. In addition, exercises are longer, with more repetitions, and often faster. All classes end with a 10-minute relaxation period based on the Mitchell Method (similar to those described on pages 143–145).

The most distinguishing features of a Bodywork class are the emphasis on increasing the student's awareness of her own body through slow deliberate exercising of every little part (hands and ankles receive attention just as much as legs and buttocks), on posture (particularly the correcting of the classic sway back syndrome), on breathing and on balance. All students are required to fill out medical forms.

Through her classes, books, teacher training courses and capacity as advisor on countless exercise projects, Barbara Dale has gone a long way towards correcting the distortions and carelessness of aerobics classes or military-style keep fit. Bodywork classes represent a redressing of the balance towards an intelligent and caring attituded to one's body. They can be recommended to all those looking for an effective body conditioning method that goes a little deeper then most, teaching you something about your body rather than just knocking it into shape.

These two methods represent two very different styles of body conditioning. We personally recommend the second type to beginners, but explore the possibilities in your area to find the right balance of work and body awareness to suit you.

Aerobics

While body conditioning and dance fitness forms of exercise have a relatively long history and are rooted in the traditions of gymnastics, yoga and dance, the recent development of so-called aerobics exercise classes is a new phenomenon, born from Kenneth Cooper's research, modified by Jacki Sorensen and stamped with glamour by Jane Fonda. Aerobics classes, though barely a decade old, have risen steeply in popularity, largely due to our desire for instant and measurable results.

The idea of converting Cooper's Aerobics Points system into a packageable routine which could be practised in the studio was Jacki Sorensen's. Already a fitness teacher, she came across Cooper's book in 1969 and set about applying his system to a dance fitness routine aimed to appeal to women. A subsequent study she conducted herself, and one done later, in 1983, by the Human Performance Laboratory at the University of Nebraska found that a 10–12 week aerobic dancing programme increased cardiovascular fitness in the unfit just as well as jogging.

Sorensen launched her programme on the public in 1971, and by 1979 had over 150,000 students over the United States. The same 'Cooper' elements appealed: the scientific basis of studies and research, the organized attention to the checking of pulse rates, the different levels of activity for different levels of fitness, and the rigidly balanced timing of every section of the class – which is not to say that aerobic dancing does not have a 'fun image'. This is stressed a great deal: lots of bounce, lots of music, and a big smile all the way through. The style is a sporty one (for the first time training shoes were required for an exercise class) with no emphasis on learning skill in movement, on suppleness or grace, or on the creative element of dance.

Because it was so simple, aerobic dancing wooed many of those women who were nervous of attending dance classes, and because it was brand new, and *fun*, it captured many clients from more regimented forms of studio exercise. Aerobic dancing as such has not come to Britain. Jacki Sorensen has patented her routine and kept within the US, but many of her techniques and style of working can be found in the aerobics classes and the newer forms of dance fitness available in Britain today.

In the late 1970s the image of studio exercise changed once again: from Sorenson's squeeky clean, all-American, ra-ra aerobic dancing (and its offshoots) to the hard-edged Hollywood glamour of Jane Fonda. Fonda's whole approach to movement and exercise has its roots in her years of ballet training and, as she candidly reveals in her *Workout* book, in the endless round of self-punishing dieting, amphetamines and living for long periods on nothing but coffee and strawberry yoghurt in the desperate attempt to conform to the slender image. Both ballet and her self-destructive regime are characterized by rigorous self-control and the exertion of will-power to achieve a goal.

Like Sorensen, Fonda adapted her past training to suit the needs, desires and capabilities of ordinary women. Asked to teach, she drew on what she knew. In this way the Fonda Workout emphasizes working to the limits of endurance, pushing the body to do more each time with the implicit aim of conforming to a set ideal. '. . . when I approach my workout', she writes, 'I am no longer Jane Fonda, the actress, wife, mother, activist. I am an athlete. I *have* to push myself to my limit and beyond because I'm preparing for competition. But the competition is with myself.'

The composition of the Workout (sometimes called the California Workout, and known in Britain by a variety of different names, usually featuring the word 'aerobic') is eclectic, drawing on yoga, jazz dance, gymnastic and ballet exercise. It is exacting and thorough, dealing with every muscle group but now moves at a fast pace making for a high risk of strain.

The actual so-called aerobic section of the California Work-out is only a maximum of 5 minutes. The fast pace of the rest of the exercises is supposed to maintain the high pulse rate. Our preference would be to go for the type of class that offered an extended 'aerobics' section (15–20 minutes) of *simple* movements done at a pace adequate for cardiovascular training, followed by stretch, toning and strength exercises done *deliberately* and at a *slow* pace. This minimises potential damage and allows you to get more satisfaction from really feeling yourself stretch, long and slowly, and from doing an exercise properly rather than skimping and rushing on to the next (see Stretching pages 115–119). But this kind of class is not, under any circumstances, for beginners. Although there is a certain divergence of opinion on the wearing of shoes in the studio, if the aerobics section is extended beyond five minutes we would advise you to wear them to cushion the jolting to joints all through the body, not just as foot protection.

There is nothing intrinsically wrong with exercising hard and fast, for women and men. And for many women this head-long plunge into blood-pounding daily workouts got them in touch with the competitive, powerful side of themselves. Their confidence in themselves and their capacity for achievement was raised. Fonda introduced the concept of competitiveness into exercise classes in a big way. The arduous aerobic workout puts speed, hard work and achievement above other criteria, such as the quality of the movement, an awareness of your body and the value of doing an exercise carefully and deliberately. This is not only misguided but potentially damaging. By going for speed and sweat it is far too easy to miss the little warning signs of strain, easy to pull a muscle or damage a joint – whether you are a beginner or a seasoned exerciser.

If you enjoy the kind of challenge and racy atmosphere of this type of class and need the pressure of competition to galvanize you into exercising, then there are plenty around to choose from. But make sure you choose a class that has a good warm-up and good cool-down period (too many teachers end their class abruptly allowing no time for the body to regulate itself and for blood to return from the muscles to the heart). Find a class where the music does not drown the instructions and where the teacher shows concern that her students perform the exercises correctly, demonstrating a knowledge of the body and pleasure in teaching.

The 'aerobics' style of exercise class is a new phenomenon with a short history, no one style or training method, no set teaching standards nor, yet, a governing body. On the whole aerobics classes cannot meet the training elements we expect from a good movement method, providing the student with a grounding in centering, control or mastery, in self-expression or developing skill, suppleness and real body awareness to enhance the mind-body collaboration. They cannot meet them because that is not their aim. Aerobics classes aim to build strength, and give some cardiovascular and flexibility training with the underlying, tacit promise and goal of increasing your attractiveness.

By all means go to an aerobics class – they can be fun and get you fitter faster than, say, a dance technique. But be aware of the limitations and the cautions. Always ask for information on a teacher's training and, once you have got yourself moving – by jumping in at the deep end – you may find you wish to progress to a movement technique which offers a deeper discipline and training.

Dance Fitness

Dance fitness classes have their foundation in dance techniques and exercise. The idea is an old one, going back (in recent history) to the early 1900s and 1920s when women began to move more freely and Isadora Duncan made her influence felt on the world of dance, encouraging flowing movement rather than technique. The links between health and dance movement began to be emphasised.

More recently the idea of fitness through dance exercise was popularized most successfully by Jacki Sorensen with her aerobic dancing. Dance exercise is a suitable way to keep fit for *all* ages and has a higher movement energy level than body conditioning, but is not as fast paced as aerobics.

There are many different dance fitness styles to choose from today and more are being created all the time. However, the basics remain much the same and can be characterized as follows: fluid, continuous routines incorporating dance steps from a variety of dance disciplines (ballet, jazz, tap, cabaret, modern); an emphasis on choreographed sequences rather than repetition of the same simple movement; continuous variety and changing pace, mood and demands, rather than intensity and build up of repetitions. Every class is likely to be different rather than a harder version of last week's. Teachers tend to come from a dance background and emphasis is on getting the exerciser to dance and use qualities of projection and creativity right from the start, but combined with circumscribed routines carefully designed to exercise every part of the body. There is no emphasis on an aerobic sequence and none on the development of a specialist technique or on strengthening a particular area of the body over and above any other. Teaching styles tend to be communicative, with lots of talking-through of the routines, explanations and corrections rather than simple mimicry of moves.

The **Medau Method** is probably the oldest and best established of the dance fitness systems still popular in Britain and even predates the Keep Fit Association by several years. Developed in Germany, the first school of Medau opened in Berlin in 1929. The founders were Heinrich Medau and his wife Senta who developed their particular form of movement exercise specifically for women after realizing that, if they exercised at all, women were merely being offered a watered-down version of men's exercises. What was needed, they felt, was something more flowing and subtle.

Teachers in Medau undergo a rigorous three year training in anatomy, physiology, choreography and music. Every Medau teacher must be able to improvize music on the piano, and while this may remind some of us of early ballet classes in draughty church halls, the effect here is quite different and an important element of the Medau method. The ability of both teacher and student to interrelate the two disciplines of music and movement, and to give shape to a movement through sound, is very enriching and takes things well beyond mere exercise. In the same way the use of balls, hoops and clubs (something also adopted by the KFA) helps to focus attention, form links between different realities (space, time, solid, void, etc) and eliminate self-consciousness and affectation. The emphasis is always on natural body movement, so there are no jerks or strenuous repetitions. Joints are not stressed, nor muscles bunched; the body is worked as a whole piece rather than in sections from the joints. Focus is put on the natural spring within the body, drawing on the tensile strength we all have. One of the basic exercises, for instance, is 'feathering', a kind of vigorous bouncing which 'stirs up' the sluggish and gets energy coursing around the body. The idea is to teach the individual to be economical with energy reserves, to learn to tap into, and coordinate, them. Medau claims to exercise students for life, not just to be able to do another class, faster and harder than the last.

You can expect to find emphasis on breathing: often in the form of wide yawns, encouraged by the teacher rather than stifled. Routines involving jumps, skips, hops and turns (the basic movements of dance with some calisthenics thrown in) are developed over the weeks. Posture is also given attention and many exercises are performed with a partner. Energy is high and a sense of fun, friendliness and cooperation are cultivated to ensure non-competitiveness.

Phyllis Morgan, founder of **Dancercise**, trained as a dancer in the USA, first with Michael Nicholoff, then at the Martha Graham School in New York. She went on to dance professionally and later became a political journalist active in the United Nations and the Peace Movement. She brings to her teaching a singularly American high energy, lots of pazazz and exacting standards; all her teachers come from dance backgrounds with good training and a high standard of performance.

Certain principles and characteristics distinguish Dancercise and it is the closest of these methods in form and vocabulary to standard dance training. All movements are fluid and flow one into the other. There is no jerking and care is taken with bouncing, particularly during the warm-up period. A certain amount of learning of new sequences (each no longer than a few linked movements) takes place in every class, both with the music, in imitation, and without the music, with verbal explanation from the teacher. Verbal encouragement is constant throughout the class; a teacher talk students through the routines in a descriptive way: so, for instance, a Dancercise teacher never counts, but rather says 'bounce, stretch, up, down, turn around' etc to mark the beat. Emphasis is on keeping the atmosphere fun and lively.

The atmosphere is non-competitive, but students are encouraged to project themselves like professional dancers and some steps are performed moving across the floor of the studio. Moving through space is an important ingredient of Dancercise (as it is in Medau) – emphasizing the exhilaration and spatial awareness of dance rather than the static quality of a keep fit class. For similar reasons – avoidance of mindless mimicry – repetition of any one step is minimal.

Each of the Dancercise teachers has a particular training and penchant, so classes reflect this: one class may concentrate on disco techniques, another on tap, a third may be stagey and performance orientated. However, the overall pattern of every class will include a warm-up session followed by 'adagio', a period of slow work to train the muscles and teach poise, balance, control. Then a faster period, full of high jumps and kicks, jazz walks and *pas chassés* across the floor, moving into floor work and slower routines for strength, and finally cool down.

Moves Fitness's creator, Cindy Gilbert, comes from the Olympic athletics back-ground rather than professional dance. Another American, from California, Cindy – all 6ft ¾ of her – was an Olympic high-jumper and pentathlete and studied kinesiology (human movement) at UCLA in the heyday of the early 1970s; new ideas about human potential were flourishing and East began to meet West to enrich our vision, not least of movement and exercise. Throughout her university years she also studied under Judi Shepherd Misset, founder of the dance fitness programme Jazzercise (only in the USA) where she learnt dance techniques, the coordination of exercise to music and above all presentation methods.

Emphasis is put on performance in the Moves Fitness teacher training, on giving to the class, projecting fun, glamour, enthusiasm. They are taught to explain, briefly, the key points of the exercises performed but essentially the class mimics the teacher. In all Moves Fitness classes four cardinal rules are emphasised and outlined: movement must always be safe, balanced, free and fun.

The routines reflect these tenets. The choreographed sequences, all designed by Cindy herself, are of uniform length (5–8 minutes) and follow symmetrical keep fit style patterns but with fluid, smooth transitions, making for continuous routines akin to short dance sequences. The pace throughout is generally up-tempo, but not furious, with a few slower routines worked in. Every class contains a collection of routines put together to exercise specifically, and in turn, all the major muscle groups of the body, combining flexes, jumping jacks, lunges, kicks and so on. The flavour is more like fluid gym than the creative irregularity of dance, but (as with Dancercise) the sequences do *not* contain repetitions, jerky, strained movements, and never rapid bounces on a stretched muscle (Cindy is vociferous on the dangers of this technique, popular in aerobics classes – see pages 112–115 for the rationale).

Just as with all exercise classes you will encounter as many different types of dance fitness as there are individual teachers. By describing the three methods above we are not trying to imply that these are the only ones worth practising. We have chosen three popular, tried and tested methods of a high standard, each significantly different in style and orientation, which are also typical of different strands of dance fitness elsewhere. They indicate what to expect and also what you should look for if you choose dance fitness as a preferred way to keep in shape. Compare your local versions of dance fitness classes with those described here.

Weight Training

Weight training is big news these days. It has supplanted running and aerobics as the latest 'in' thing in the exercise world. Hollywood stars, business executives, housewives as well as 8-stone weaklings are all taking it up with a passion which matches the zeal of the born-again-runners from the halcyon days of jogging. Yet as a form of physical training it has been in existence as long as any of our other major sports.

There are two threads which run through the history of

weight training. One is training for power and strength in order to improve performance in a given sport or activity; the other is training for aesthetics: bodybuilding à la Mr Universe and Mr Olympia competitions. This is an important distinction in terms of your goals.

Nineteenth century Europe saw the emergence of systematic weight training. Friedrich Ludwig Jahn, instrumental in initiating physical training regimes in Prussia, found that some of his students were not strong enough to perform his gymnastic exercises and so introduced a variety of weights for his students to improve their strength first. But some of his students became more interested in the weight training and clubs were set up all over Germany. Louis Attila, born in 1844 in Baden Baden, trained at one of these clubs. He was a professional strong man who performed his feats all over Europe. He became so famous that in 1887 he was selected to perform at Queen Victoria's Golden Jubilee and was subsequently presented at Court. But it was with his even more famous student, Eugene Sandow, who popularized the use of dumb-bells during his act, that weight lifting, as we know it, was born. Sandow had one other asset: he was physically very beautiful. Suddenly the muscle-and-moustaches strong man was out of fashion. The body beautiful was in vogue, and in 1898 Bernard MacFadden started the magazine *Physical Culture*. Five years later, in 1903, the first Physical Culture Competition was held in Madison Square Garden in New York City.

Since then we have seen the continued commercialization of bodybuilding. There have been a large number of different organizations established, all laying claim to being the governing body of weight training, but there are two which stand out. The International Federation of Body Builders, which is based in Montreal, sponsors the Mr Olympia competition. In Britain the 25-year-old National Amateur British Bodybuilding Association is well-established and sponsors the Mr Universe competition. Both of these organizations focus on bodybuilding.

The British Amateur Weight Lifting Association is the best source of information on weight training. During its early days it met with suspicion due to the ignorance of most of the national sports coaches as to the value of weights, and because of confusion with the bodybuilding image to which it had

erroneously become connected. But some far-sighted individuals like Dan Maskell of tennis fame, Walter Winter-
bottom, coaching director of the Football Association, and the
armed services PT schools encouraged the use of weight
training techniques to the advantage of their athletes. The
increased recognition of the training effects of strength training
has led to weight training now being more universally applied
than any other form on physical training. Once the province
of the executive, the professional body builder, or the wimp
aspiring to Atlas stature, gyms are now also host to women eager
to try their hand at pumping iron. As ordinary women began to
expose their bodies in sport and physical training rather than in
Playboy magazines and Pirelli calendars, it was seen that women
did possess muscles. The initial novelty and shock value of this
phenomenon was broken to the public by body builder Lisa
Lyon and others giving voice and exposure to their pursuits.
Female body builders began to come out of the closet. Whether
you are a body builder, a sprinter, a ballet dancer, a karateka, or
simply recovering from an injury, weight training is an essential
aspect of development.

In order to train effectively with weights, it is important to
have some basic knowledge of anatomy. All weight training is
muscle specific, so you need to know which ones you are going
to train. In addition you need to know when to train with
'specific exercises', in order to isolate a muscle for strengthening, or 'massive exercises' for training entire muscle groups.
You should have some idea of the advantage of 'single set
systems', 'multiple set systems' and 'flushing systems'.

Single set systems consist of one set of repetitions prescribed
for a particular muscle or muscle group. The number of repetitions may start small and build up to twelve or more.
Multiple set systems use heavier weights and fewer repetitions in a
set. But the individual may employ as many as 10 sets for
maximizing power development. *Flushing systems* involve using
sets of different exercises which all focus in a different way on
the same muscle or muscle group. The buildup results in the
muscles being 'flushed' with blood. Isotonic, isometric, isokinetic and variable resistance training techniques are all important aspects of proper training. These aspects of strength
training are touched upon in the section on Strength in Physical
Goals (see pages 93–100), but a serious pursuit of weight training

will require more extensive research.

Because of the amount of weight being used and the specific physical goals usually pursued in weight training, it is very important to do it *right*. Injuries due to misuse and stupidity (which often includes a large percentage of ego) are common, but increasingly proper supervision is reducing the injuries caused by ignorance. One of the key factors in choosing a gym is the amount of supervision and care you receive. It is not enough to be simply left alone to sort it out yourself. This is one reason why the Pilates technique (page 281) is so recommended by us: there is a high degree of personal and caring supervision. Demand qualified, individual attention, or find somewhere else that will provide it. 'Buddy' systems are very common in weight training clubs. As you progress in your experience and goals, there are a variety of exercises and situations which require assistance from a friend.

Weight training can be used as a complementary activity to whatever your primary sport might be. Because of the different kinds of weight, set, repetition, sequencing and muscle specific exercises, it is possible to train with weights for any physical activity you choose. Bodybuilding works specifically for moulding and shaping your body for aesthetic reasons, but if you want to improve your performance in your tennis or your judo or your modern dance, get in touch with the BAWLA to find out how you can develop a training regime which meets the specific needs of your activity.

Choosing between training equipment is not easy. Before the exercise boom, there were only free weights: barbells and dumb-bells. More equipment was introduced like squat stands, flat benches, dead lift exercisers, incline benches, leg extensor machines, etc, which incorporate pulleys and cables to increase the range of possible exercises. Someone then got the idea to put them all together and the Multi Gym, or Universal Gym, was born: a collection of twelve or more exercise stations built into a central framework which allow an individual to travel around practising one exercise after another.

Enter Arnold Jones and his revolutionary Nautilus equipment – as exercise physiologist Tony Lycholat says: 'now as well-known in the fitness world as Hoover is in the land of carpet cleaning'. Unlike free weights, the Nautilus equipment is designed to make the same demands upon a muscle from the beginning to the end of its range of movement. Jones utilized the cam mechanism to achieve this, and the Nautilus boom was born. Nowadays there is a slight backlash against Nautilus-type equipment and, generally speaking, there is widespread agreement amongst unbiased experts that weight training should incorporate a variety of approaches rather than just isokinetic variable resistance machines like Nautilus. Dumb-bells and barbells are back in vogue! In any event it is as well to be aware that in addition to Nautilus there are Atlanta, Hydrafitness, David, Polaris, Schnell and Nissen, to mention a few of the more common makes of equipment of this type. All have advantages and disadvantages to be explored.

There is no doubt that weight training gives you a sense of both self-mastery and a genuine sense of achievement. There are such obvious goals and such clear pathways to achieve them. While sometimes accused of undue narcissism, this concentration on one's body can be turned into self-exploration. In addition, if you have ever watched a bodybuilding competition you will know that there is a definite quotient of artistry in the presentation of the participants.

The one great drawback of weight training is that it is so specific to strength training goals. Weight training should include flexibility exercises and neuromuscular coordination techniques as well. On its own weight training will eventually lead to a restricted range of motion of the joints, a reduction in speed and fine motor coordination. Train for other physical goals to complement weight training and the result will be a more balanced cultivation of overall physical well being.

Circuit Training

Circuit training is probably the most common training regime used by a wide range of sports and activities in order to improve performance. A circuit consists of a number of different stations at which the athlete performs a given exercise as many times as is possible within a given time period. When the time is completed the individual moves on to the next station and performs a different exercise for a similar period of time and so on around the various stations. Upon completion of a circuit the individual may rest or begin a repetition of the same circuit. Circuit training can be designed to increase a variety of physical qualities including muscular strength, flexibility, muscular endurance, and cardiovascular fitness.

A circuit should be designed around the aspect of his performance the individual is seeking to improve. If it is primarily strength you are interested in, then a circuit will include weight resistance exercises – in fact, most weight training and body building routines are variations of circuit training regimes. If you are mainly concerned with an endurance activity then you may want to include a variety of running, swimming or cycling exercises in your circuit. These will improve cardiovascular fitness as well as provide endurance training for the muscles.

But the true advantage of circuit training lies in the wide mixture of training techniques which can be incorporated. As well as a variety of exercises using equipment it is possible to incorporate exercises like sit-ups, squats, pull ups and also sprints, runs, swimming pool lengths, etc. In addition a variety of exercises directed at overcoming a specific weakness can be incorporated into a generl training circuit for your sport. Exercises for flexibility and range of movement can also be included, and would play an important part in a warming-up session for ballet or for a martial art like tae kwon do which requires considerable hip flexibility. As a result of this adaptability a circuit can be designed which will meet not only the needs of your activity (be it martial arts, dancing or another body conditioning system) but will also help you to train those parts of yourself which are not up to the standards required by your particular activity.

There are a number of guidelines which are followed when setting up a circuit. The stations are usually between eight and fifteen in number, and will take anywhere from five to twenty minutes to complete. Very often the stations are organized in a circular fashion so that you can progress smoothly from one station to the next. The sequence of the exercise is organized so that you don't usually train the same muscle group on consecutive stations; muscles are thus trained more completely and there is less work on the ehart and circulatory system. Exercises are done to a set time limit, usually of either 30 seconds or 60 seconds, and during this time the participant is meant to produce as many repetitions as possible. With some endurance exercises, the factor is speed or, as with a cycling machine, the number of wheel revolutions. At the end of each station, the individual should be near fatigue in that particular muscle group. Limited rest is allowed between stations: 15 to 20 seconds is common. As with many training systems, the principle of progressive overload should be met. Periodical increases in weight, resistance, time and reductions in rest intervals will help maintain overload. In the course of a training session you may expect to complete a circuit more than once, three times being common.

The variety of possible circuits is limitless. Following the above guidelines and information from training texts on the specific exercises commonly used in circuit training, you can build up your own circuit or, with the advice of a coach, trainer or physiotherapist, set up circuits which will provide a comprehensive training regime which can be regularly varied. In this way you can systematically train your body. It will help to reduce training boredom if you are creative and innovative with your mixture of stations and training systems. The only caveat (as with any training system which is self-administered and regulated) is to make certain that you don't injure yourself through improper execution of the recommended exercises. Don't overdo a good thing.

Dance

Dance for recreation and fitness has seen a revival over the last exercise-hooked decade. Encouraged by the urge to move, people have started to explore beyond the aerobics field and the gym, finding that the tried and tested dance forms have much to offer as recreation and a stimulating way to keep in shape. Forms as varied as ballet, tap, Humphrey and Chantraine are now enjoying a new and steady flow of interest. They deserve to be explored further.

Dance is where movement and art meet, it is a form in which every individual can experience his creativity immediately, through the body, in the satisfying knowledge that he is part of a tradition that stretches back into the past, and part of a living, changing art form that will continue to evolve in the future.

Dance appeals to the mind, the spirit and the emotions, allowing us to experience these parts of ourselves together through the whole of our body; and not just experience but express – joy, sadness, fun, exhilaration, anger. Fitness is not just about moving muscles and raising the heart rate to a certain level. It is a sense of well being and it is about feeling more alive, experiencing all the parts of oneself living in harmony. Dance is, as all societies have known, one of the very best vehicles for making this vitality a regular part of our lives.

The beauty of dance is that anyone can do it and you don't have to go to classes or have lessons. When we dance at a party or go to a disco we don't think about how fit we're getting – we have a good time. The fact that we may work up a good sweat and increase the flexibility of our joints is an unconsidered plus – the main factor is that we feel excited, glowing, letting the music dictate our body's movements and rhythm. Dance scores high on the well being stakes!

The spontaneous reaction of people throughout the ages and across the cultures to certain rhythms and beats is to dance. And even in the more restrained countries of Europe and America, dance crazes have gripped the popular imagination and swept everyone along in a fever of excitement. The waltz, the Charleston, the Lindy, jive and jitterbug, Rock 'n' Roll, the Twist, Soul and disco – popular styles have come and gone. They have always developed hand in hand with the popular music of the time, have always been part of the youth culture and have always had an explosive effect on the society of the day, with implications beyond their recreative value.

The Lindy, for example, developed during the Depression of the 1930s in America. At one of the dance marathons where young couples danced for days in the hope of winning huge prize money, a young black, in an effort to vary the monotony, broke away from his partner and improvised upon a little known dance called the Lindy, thus bringing it to public attention. This new version was smoothly violent, suffused with the grim irony of those hard times. Innovative because it shifted dance away from the couple formation, the Lindy was soon adopted by white America, danced to the mellower sounds of Swing and dubbed the Jitterbug. It was the precursor of jive in the USA and of the British version, Rock 'n' Roll. It was during this intense period when dance was caught up with the racial and social conflicts of black and white, of youth and authority, that a real gymnastic element entered popular dance styles, to remain through the styles of the 60s, 70s and 80s.

Television helped to fan the flame of the dance explosion started by Bill Haley and his 'Rock Around the Clock' and continued through such American stars as Buddy Holly, Little Richard and Elvis Presley. Rock 'n' Roll was a particularly teenage phenomenon, since the kids of the 50s had more money to spend, and with 'Elvis the Pelvis' sex was explicitly re-introduced, setting of the mass hysteria that became such a feature of beatlemania and the rock concerts of the 1960s.

Although popular dancing hit an all time low in the 60s when psychodelorama and spectacular stage shows took over from the more intimate relationship between dancer and music, old styles, like Rock 'n' Roll, or going further back, the Tango, Charleston, Samba and others have not been lost. These and others are now enjoying a revival as people's imaginations are caught by the colour and energy of these different dance languages. Folk dances, eastern, Kathakali or belly dancing, Scottish and Irish reels, Morris and clog dancing, these and many other ancient traditional dance forms are gaining fresh attention from those attracted to an earlier heritage. The choice today is vast.

Venues, have changed over the last decade. It is now the exception rather than the rule to learn and practise your favourite dance steps on Friday night at the local dance hall, whether it be Latin American or jive. As space became more expensive so the large dance halls were replaced by the small night-club or discotheque, the cramped areas giving rise, incidentally, to more restricted dance styles (like the up-and-down movements of disco and the Pogo). The opening during the 1970s of the large dance studios was due in large part to the cost and overcrowding in these fashionable clubs. Studios like the Dance Centre, the Urdang and then the Pineapple, all in London, provided large rooms where people could learn to dance, and for the first time the lay person who loved to dance was rubbing shoulders with the professional. This helped inspire the growth of interest among the public in the techniques of dance; methodology, styles and practice routines tended to dominate over spontaneous fun and expression, fuelled also by the fitness boom and the close proximity of the gym and the workout class.

The tide is beginning to turn somewhat now and dance teachers are recognizing that it is important to bring back the expressive and spontaneous if people are to be encouraged to *enjoy* dancing.

In the West we tend to assume that dance classes are only for the dedicated and the specialist. Too often we equate dance lessons with ballet (if you didn't start at five years old, don't bother), or with modern dance (you need legs six feet long and must sport pink leg warmers), or with ballroom (old-fashioned and you need a dedicated mother to sew on the sequins). But of course our assumptions need only apply to those who wish to make a serious career out of dance. For the rest of us learning to dance at an amateur level can be immensely fulfilling. And in the hands of a gifted teacher, you can expect to find it satisfying from the very first class. In the first instance this is because your mind and your imagination are engaged. You concentrate on learning movements, techniques, shapes, rhythms, styles and in the process can forget yourself and the worries of daily life.

In the next stage you experience the pleasure of mastering a skill, of gaining a vocabulary and seeing your body respond and adapt to this new language. And in the third stage you learn to express yourself in this new form. Of course these stages in the learning process overlap and a good teacher will encourage expression and an awareness of the sheer joy of dancing from the very beginning.

In the following sections we take a look at some of the standard dance forms like jazz and ballet which you can expect to find taught in classes. In addition we describe some newer forms like Contact Improvisation and Chantraine, which are less well known but have much to offer the individual who wants to discover the body's expression through music but is less interested in mastering the skill of a complex technique.

These newer forms have developed from diverse roots but they also share the influence of the more general trends, such as the growth of feminism and a concern with more holistic approaches to life, that underlie a great many of the movement forms we describe in this book, and Stage Two Fitness in general.

The emphasis in contemporary dance on the individual's experience and relationship with the body as being of equal value to the aesthetics of performance, is grounded in a long-standing and still developing area of dance, that of dance-movement therapy. Certain pioneers, like Rudolph von Laban, Lulu Sweigard and Margaret Morris, among many others, recognized the creative potential for the lay person in dance. Their contribution to our contemporary perception of dance and our participation has been far-reaching, and their seminal work has crossed more barriers than just those of the worlds of dance and therapy.

Laban, born in Hungary in the late nineteenth century, was one of the mainsprings behind the dance revolution in Europe and America during the first half of this century. A choreographer, Laban developed new ways of looking at human movement, and of making dance accessible to everyone, not just the professionals. He devised a classification system of human movement, and later a notation system which are still used throughout the world, both in dance and in psychology. He analysed movement as conditioned by the structure of the body and space, and showed that the dynamism in movement stems from the different kinds of control in the release of human energy. In 1910 he founded the first group of non-professional dancers in Berlin. He moved to Britain in the 1930s where his ideas were applied in a diversity of fields – dance, theatre, therapy, and the industrial and educational sectors. His influence has been profound and the Laban Centre, part of the University of London's Goldsmiths' College, continues to teach his principles and ideas in a variety of classes, courses and workshops, primarily for professional dancers and teachers.

While Laban is a household name in the world of dance, few today have heard of Margaret Morris. Her influence has, however, been significant. Trained as a ballerina, she rebelled against the artificialities of the Italian ballet and began to evolve her own dance technique. This was consolidated after studying with Isadora Duncan's brother from whom she learned the Greek positions he had reconstructed from murals and vases. These basic positions which emphasised the natural opposition of limbs became the key movements in the system now known as Margaret Morris Movement. In 1910 she opened a school, one of the first to teach dance and movement for recreation and pleasure rather than for performance. Noticing the beneficial effects on her pupils' health, she became more interested in the therapeutic potential of movement and trained as a physiotherapist at St. Thomas's Hospital, London, which then adopted her creative movement system into its remedial department. She also devised a system of movement notation. In 1937, she was one of the founding members of the National Council for Physical Fitness, and in 1960 she founded the Scottish National Ballet.

There are now MMM centres worldwide and the organization continues to promote the concept of movement as creative, a balance between technique, improvisation and free expression, designed specifically for the non-professional.

Another similar system of dance created by ex-dancers and aimed at the non-professional is the Chantraine Method, described more fully on pages 236–238). This is where dance meets movement for health, and both these systems successfully combine the two worlds of exercise and dance.

The Association for Dance Movement Therapy was founded in 1981 by ex-dancers keen to extend their usefulness as dancers beyond the few years of a professional career. They work with the emotionally disturbed and the physically disabled, within the social services and with psychologists and psychiatrists. They also run workshops open to anyone interested in expanding their experience of dance.

More and more psychotherapists are acknowledging the prime importance of movement and body awareness to psychological and emotional health. Rather than being considered a hobby or leisure pursuit dance and creative physical expression are fast becoming vital elements in the emerging holistic approach to fitness. Some of the myths surrounding dance are dropping away as well. It is no longer a female preserve populated by the lithe and fragily graceful ballerinas interspersed with the odd Nureyev, all muscled thighs and silent strength.

The relationship between movement and music is dance's crucial offering to the richness of our life and our well being. No other movement form offers us quite this opportunity to both learn and strive for a skill while expressing the creativity which springs from our innate gifts and our experience in the world. The balance between technique and art is a special one and can have enriching repercussions on the way we live the rest of our lives.

Ballet

Ballet holds an attraction for both dancers and spectators, for young and old, women and men, second to none in the world of dance. In city centres, theatres, school stages and church halls ballet continues to cast its magic spell.

The history of ballet is a long and fascinating one, as it developed from its origins in the French courtly dances of the sixteenth century via the codifying era of the eighteenth century, the golden age of Romanticism, the brilliance and rigid training of the Russian system to the diversification of the twentieth century. It is also a history of individuals, such as Pierre Beauchamps who formulated the five basic ballet positions, Carlo Blasis who codified the ballet and laid down rules for training. Marie Taglioni, the Romantic prima donna who is credited as the first to dance en pointe, Enrico Cecchetti whose method trained some of the greatest Russian stars, and all those other names from Pavlova to Baryshnikov which have given ballet an almost mythical place in our culture.

In the twentieth century, and particularly in recent decades there have been revolts against this rigidly controlled, 'unrealistic' dance form. A lot of choreographers have brought ballet into modern times by incorporating ideas and techniques from modern dance, and by moving away in their subject matter from the romanticism of such ballets as *Swan Lake* and *La Sulphide*. However, the classical training remains supreme in dance for its thoroughness, its meticulousness and its ability to build tremendous strength and explosive power combined with a smooth and seemingy effortless execution. Most of the top modern dancers either studied ballet when young or turned to it later to refine their skill.

The perennial appeal of ballet to the non-professional who wishes to dance for pleasure an drecretion lies in its romantic and glamorous image – only Hollywood or the rock music world can rival ballet for the galaxy of stars it produces. And only ballet stars earn the adulation of their public through the unique combination of gruelling hard work, total dedication to their art and the ability to make it all seem effortless, graceful, belonging to another world. The essence of ballet comes to us from the age of Romanticism, the first half of the nineteenth century, when the ballerina came to be glorified and the male dancer relegated to a secondary, supporting role, the ballerina represented the archetypal romantic woman: enchanting, delicate, graceful yet with inner strength and will and, above all, unattainable. The gauze and tulle and floating tissues of ballet costume were first used during this era: they emphasized the evanescent and ethereal quality of this ideal creature. The robustness of earlier times, when male stars were admired for their technical virtuosity, was only brought back into ballet with the great Russian male stars of this century.

Ballet's appeal for someone wishing to dance does not lie solely in its dreamy escapist images. The development of ballet technique over the centuries has led to great refinement of a very powerful expressive vocabulary. It was Michel Fokine, the Russian choreographer working with Diaghilev in Paris, who emphasized the expressive nature of ballet and eliminated the pantomime element and ornamental additions from the dance. Instead the entire body should express significant movement: 'man can be and should be expressive from head to foot'. The language of ballet is sophisticated and subtle and there can be immense satisfaction in learning it. The rigour and exactness of the training concentrates the mind and disciplines the body, but the moment of dance comes with the ability to transcend the strict vocabulary of codified movements and infuse it with personal expression. It is this that contributes to the genius of Nureyev or Pavlova, and it is these models of supreme achievement that the student has in mind as inspiration during the hard work of training.

Ballet is based on an artificial use of the body. While this is true to a certain extent for any dance form or sport, since anything practised consistently over a long period of time will shape the body to conform to the effort, it is more true for ballet than for anything else. For the young girl pursuing ballet as a profession the dangers of striving to conform to the idealized image of the ballerina against the natural growth of the body can result in disillusionment, disturbed eating habits and finally, for many, a sense of failure. Men are not affected in this way, although the male ideals exert their own pressure. However, the person choosing ballet as a form of recreation and exercise need not be affected by these problems and can enjoy the rigour of the dance form without taking on board its pitfalls.

The correct stance in ballet is with spine erect, rib cage expanded and pulled upward with all the strength coming from tight stomach and buttock muscles. All movement in ballet is based on what is known as the turnout. This ideally 180 degree turnout of the legs starts from the hips and takes years of hard work to achieve. It was introduced in the late seventeenth century when performances moved from the round in private courts to the raised and sloped stages of the public theatres. Since the show could now only be seen from the front, intricate floor patterns were lost to the spectator, and instead the movements themselves became more important. Dancers were forced to move from side to side and in order to do so gracefully the turnout was developed. This also enabled the dancer to perform brilliant leaps and turns. Unnatural though it may feel, the turnout is still the foundation of classical ballet.

There are five basic positions, all founded on the turnout,

from which all movement springs; these positions, in various different forms, define the official poses in ballet. There are seven prescribed ways to move in classical ballet, always known by their French names, such as: plier (to bend), étendre (to stretch), etc, and it is when these movements and positions are combined that they become dance. The beginner, however, will spend most of the time learning basic techniques before combining the positions with movement in short sequences.

Correct body placement is constantly stressed in ballet, and great emphasis is put in training on visual self-correction – hence the large floor to ceiling mirrors. The effect in performance rather than the dancer's experience is everything in ballet.

Every class starts with work at the barre. The barre provides the necessary support so that the student can push her body that much further. The extended positions in ballet could never be achieved without this resistance to work against. Exercises are always done alternately and in opposition: the aim is to build strength without muscle bulk. Consequently there are few repetitions in ballet and a bend will be followed by a stretching or lifting movement, big, extended lines will be succeeded by exercises involving shorter, sharper movements.

Ballet works the legs, feet and hip joints to a maximum that you will not find in any other form of dance, and nowhere is precision so insisted upon as in the classical training. Because the turnout is so difficult, dancers are tempted to fake or cheat with small adjustments of knee and foot. A good teacher is vigilant in forbidding such practices, since this can easily lead to injury later when the strain of full body weight in complex movement could damage muscles and joints which are not correctly placed.

For the beginner ballet offers a rich and illustrious tradition, it offers discipline, structure and the pleasure of achievement step by step. For those who are self-conscious in free form movement this is very rewarding.

Jazz and Tap Dance

Jazz dance has its roots in the Black American culture which developed from the slave plantations in the deep South from the seventeenth century. Because of these origins the popular image of jazz dance is sensual, earthy, and often raw or primal. It can be all these things and has certainly retained the full-blooded energy of its creators. However, modern jazz has an inbuilt versatility which lends itself to a great range of creative expression from the sensuous to the abstract or conceptual. Confusion exists because jazz dance is most commonly seen in its popularized, cruder forms in cabaret, musicals and on television; rarely do we get to see modern dance in its richer, truly creative form as developed by a few great choreographers such as Jack Cole, Matt Mattox, Luigi or the better known Bob Fosse.

Generations of American Blacks created new dances from old tribal rhythms, overlaid by steps and sequences picked up from other immigrants to enrich their dances. Rhythms were sensuous, fluid, rich with subdued violence, reflecting the tensions of their situation. In the 1920s much innovative energy came from the Harlem district of New York where the Black population would dance in the ballrooms of 'jook' houses (an anglicized version of *dzuga* – wicked – and probably the origin of our juke boxes). White entrepreneurs introduced the risqué dances in well-packaged shows downtown, the white audience learned the dances in watered-down versions and a new dance craze swept the country. In the 1920s the effects on social convention were radical. Flappers bobbed their hair, raised their skirts, swung their pearls to the Charleston and demanded the vote. The jazz age was born.

In jazz music and dance grew hand in hand. Many of the early tunes have dance titles: the stomp, the rag, the shuffle and the Charleston. Swing, the big band sound which followed Rhythm 'n' Blues, was a movement of the arms before it became a musical catchword. The sweet sound of swing, as epitomized by Benny Goodman, was developed very much as the white answer to the earthier undertones of black jazz, altogether too threatening to a rabidly racist America. Not an exclusively white phenomenon, however, there were some internationally famous black swing bands too, like Duke Ellington and Count Basie. But the general effect was a slickening-up of both the music and the dances, with the disturbing undercurrents ironed out.

The assimilation of jazz into the mainstream was continued in the era of the Hollywood musical when stars like Fred Astaire and Ginger Rogers combined ballroom with gymnastics, tango with tap and enthralled millions. The roots once more are in black jazz: Astaire was coached by a great but now little known black choreographer, Buddy Bradley, to whom we owe most of the forms in modern jazz dance.

Tap dance is a form of jazz dance, that developed in an eclectic way via the touring minstrel shows of the turn of the century to reach a pinnacle of popularity with the Hollywood musicals of the 1930s and 40s.

Tap's appeal is obvious and immediate. Uncomplicated in terms of expression, it is snappy and witty, humorous and relaxed, and, at its best, lends itelf to wonderfully breathtaking feats of skill and acrobatics.

Tap has its origins in English clog dancing and the Irish jig. The Black slaves were exposed to these dance forms on the plantations but it was not until after the Civil War in 1854 that, with the great influx of Irish immigrants, the freed slaves, now struggling to make their way alongside the Irish poor, really began to experiment with the fast-moving jig. The Negroes added their own particular way of moving – loose limbed, curled over into a crouching position with both knees well bent – to the fancy, on-the-spot footwork of the jig. This kind of dancing, which also had a lot of the African stomp in it, came to be known as jigging. Music was provided with whatever could be mustered, with everyone joining in and creating complex improvisations and poly-rhythms around the basic tune. This was in effect the first jazz dancing. Another important precursor of tap was 'patting Juba' – the stamping, patting, clapping noises which had been a part of Black American dancing from the days the plantation owners confiscated the rousing drums from their African slaves for fear of trouble.

In the mid 1800s a certain Master Juba, a skilled tap dancer and sought after for performances, added another essential stylistic element to tap. He split the body in half. Until then the whole, and particularly the middle, body was used in dance, and in the strand of this early form that developed into modern jazz dancing this continued to be the case. But Juba stopped using the upper body and concentrated all energy into complex rhythms and patterning of the legs and feet. This tap style remained in favour up to the 1930s, when more showy techniques and acrobatic virtuosity were demanded by Hollywood. But it still characterizes the American style of tap: relaxed, lots of shuffle, complicated steps with arms loose at the sides or making the odd flapping gesture. Certain styles emerged, such as the Soft Shoe – the hat and cane routine which is a mixture of walking and shuffling so familiar from the Broadway musical. Steel taps, making for a crisper sound, came in around the 1930s. English tap is lighter, slicker, with arms performing complementary movements as in ballet. You see both kinds used in shows and musicals.

Eclecticism has always been a vital part of jazz because it is essentially an improvisational form. Like the jazz musician, the jazz dancer improvizes on and around the basic tune or steps, drawing on whatever seems meaningful and relevant, to create a uniquely energized style.

Jazz dance retains the stomping, thumping feet movements from West African tribal dances, and the earthiness of ground-orientated stances such as the loose bent knee posture, and movements like the ripple through the body from floor to skull. But they are combined with the lighter, intricate step patterns from Irish jigs, the English square dance or French quadrille. Elements from the famous social dances of the 1920s and 30s – the Charleston, the Lindy – can be traced in the jazz singer's vocabulary, too. The finger clicking and high-flung arms come from the Spanish flamenco. Oriental elements were added to the basic African rhythms by the 'father' of modern jazz, Jack Cole, who, as a student at Denishawn learnt yoga and Indian dance styles.

In the 1950s Black musicians introduced Be-Bop, a deliberate attempt to reclaim what they felt to be their sound from the sugared tones and degeneration into merely commercial dance music that swing had become. Be-Bop, with its complex phrasing and unpredictable, changeable rhythms, was undanceable. Jazz dancing went underground to re-emerge later, via choreographers like Cole, Jerome Robbins, Matt Mattox and others, as the more technically structured form we know as modern jazz.

What are the results of this mixed background? A style of dance that is vital, propulsive and acrobatic, using wide spaces and large gestures; but a style that is also subtle and lyrical; jazz dance is raw, explosive or smooth and percussive, it is both driving and insistent yet relaxed in its informality. All movement originates from the solar plexus giving it a highly charged character. Breadth and width are stressed more than height and verticality in jazz dance through the broad base provided by the wide stance of the legs. In a passage from *Total Education in Ethnic Dance* (1977), La Meri indicates the importance the spine has in jazz:

> Without the control of the spine all mastery of the technique of the limbs is without flavour. The very lift of a leg changes character completely by the placement of the lower spine. The spine is the emotional thermometer . . . The spine line shows not only immediate moods but also the mood character of a race.

Teacher/choreographers such as Luigi and Matt Mattox developed standard exercises and formulated jazz techniques which have now been taught and disseminated in the United States and Europe. This will form the basis of any class with the rest made up by the individual teacher – in the improvisational tradition of jazz. However, the majority of jazz teachers come from a show dance or television background, and the class is unlikely to reflect the depth and precision demanded by the masters. Jazz dance offers the lay person something quite distinct from other forms: the vitality and sensuous quality which stems from its ethnic roots plus the opportunity to improvise using a wide vocabulary of movements and techniques from the stomp to the most subtle of foot or arm movements.

Modern Dance

Ballet's hegemony in the world of dance began to be seriously challenged from the turn of the century, principally in America and Germany. Isadora Duncan showed that barefoot could be graceful; explorations into oriental, folk and tribal dance made themselves felt; and the research of physiologists and movement therapists into function and flow was picked up. All these things began to have their effect on the art of dance in the West.

Like the Renaissance studio tradition modern dance grew on a system of apprenticeship. This made for a rich, varied but continuous development of creative expression, with new forms grafted on to original techniques. Even today, dancers of the Humphrey or Graham techniques can trace themselves back via a distinguished lineage to the originators. This organic development is intrinsic to the character of modern dance itself.

Like modern art, modern dance has been concerned to model not *from* life but *out* of life, and not to make a facsimile but an equivalent expression. It was also concerned to use the body to a fuller capacity, to create dance out of the body's natural movements rather than to use it to portray a story, as has been the tradition in classical ballet. The general concern of the pioneers was to delve into fundamentals and the very essence of the inner life of humankind, to disclose basic truths and realities.

Modern dance techniques developed out of the need for innovation, and were inspired by creative dancers who broke the accepted mode of classical ballet. Isadora Duncan began her dancing career with Loie Fuller, who had captivated Paris with her wild, flowing dances using lights and long swathes of diaphanous material dyed in radium salts for extraordinary effects. Duncan was the first to do away with the ballet slipper and establish the bare foot in dance. She danced to music by modern and classical composers rather than dance tunes (an innovation initiated by Diaghilev with the Ballet Russe in collaboration with composers like Eric Satie). Duncan created something quite unique from her visions of Ancient Greece. Her movement was undisciplined, free flowing, sensuous and exuberant. And, perhaps more importantly, she showed Americans that *Americans* could dance. One of the inhibitions that had always dogged American culture was their sense of inferiority in the arts in relation to Europe – Duncan gave them confidence to express themselves and initiate in this new area.

The second foundation for modern dance was the Denishawn School (1915–1932, first in Los Angeles, lastly in New York), founded by the dancers Ruth St Denis and her husband Ted Shawn. They were among the first to explore and incorporate into their choreography oriental and classical dance, but their greater importance was in providing a seminal training ground for the students who trained with them. Denishawn demanded allegiance and inspired fruitful rebellion. Martha Graham, Doris Humphrey and Charles Weidman were all Denishawn pupils.

The third influence was that of German Expressionism. Mary Wigman was a German dancer who brought to America the darkness and sense of tragedy from a war-torn Europe. She provided a counterpoint to Duncan's exuberance, bringing weight and the orderliness of the Teutonic tradition. Her use of space and the use of improvisation as a teaching tool were reinforced by other important German figures: Rudolph von Laban and later the dancer Hanya Holm, a pupil of Wigman, who founded a school in New York based on her teacher's ideas.

Martha Graham is one of the best known names in modern dance. In 1923 she left Denishawn to choreograph and perform solos, later founding a small company of women dancers. A pioneer, she gained a cult following and eventually a large public.

Graham said of the early days spent developing her technique that she sought 'significant movement':

> I did not want it to be beautiful or fluid. I wanted it to be fraught with inner meaning, excitement and surge. I wanted to lose the facile quality. I did not want it to leak out, so I concentrated in a small space.

The emotional tenor of her dancing reflected this intensity, concerned as it was with dramatizing experience, extracting the essence from the meaning of her subject matter. The subjects of the Graham repertoire suited the intensity of her style. They were drawn from barbaric-primitive themes, pagan or early Christian, Puritanism, the American experience and ideals, ancient Greek myths, the experience of women.

Graham's work had a vigorous physicality. One of her earliest innovations was to use the drumming of bare feet across the boards of the stage as an insistent and disturbing rhythm. Her aim was for straightforward movement forcefully expressed. In her early work Graham made no attempt to hide the effort involved in dancing, and from the start she showed the energy of her dance in the most direct way she knew. This resulted in an aggressive, primitive style, angular and percussive. A curl, for instance, would be sudden, expressive of violence rather than of soft receptivity. Economy of movement is always valued in the Graham technique.

Graham technique evolved out of a continual search for a new movement language. Movements now used in classes often came from choreography and vice versa. There are a number of set technical exercises which must be mastered. The Graham class always begins with floorwork (about 45 minutes). This corresponds to the barre work done at the start of a ballet class. Here preparations are made for the contractions – which is in effect a lengthening of the back. The movements are small at first to warm the back and pelvis. (the source of all movement) and to prepare also for the spiral, which is the basis of all turns in Graham.

From simple beginnings complex sequences are built up on the floor, including work done on the knees. Once standing, exercises are carried out not only in all the ballet positions, but also in parallel. Great attention is paid to placement and the barre is often used. As well as 'brushes', high beats and pliés, there are special exercises unique to Graham, such as the knee vibrations, and the falls from a standing position.

For those who want to explore serious thematic dance and the ability of movement to express universal pre-occupations, Graham has a great deal to offer. The style also builds great physical strength, particularly in the muscles of the back and abdominal area, although, if it is badly taught, it is also the lower back and hip area that will be liable to strain.

A choreographer of enormous distinction, Graham created a style and an art, and her teaching techniques still form the basis for many general modern dance classes.

Doris Humphrey broke away from the Denishawn School in the late 1920s by mutual agreement: she was too radical and too purist for their liking, and the school was too eclectic and compromising for hers.

With her partner, Charles Weidman, who provided a fruitful counterpoint of wit, humour and a talent for improvisation and everyday gesture, Humphrey founded first a dance company then, in 1928, the Humphrey-Weidman School in New York. It was the first American modern dance company for both men and women and Ted Shawn's Denishawn initiatives of choreographing male solos and male group dances were developed to provide men with the opportunity to perform as dancers in their own right rather than in the limited partnering role offered at that time by classical ballet.

Doris Humphrey's aim was to find a truly indigenous form of expression in dance, one that sprang from the American experience and traditions. She wanted to bring dance closer to people and their daily lives, to abandon the fictitious and get to the root of the matter.

At the base of the Humphrey style is the principle of fall and recovery, a theory of movement fully developed by Humphrey after reading Nietzche's *Birth of Tragedy*. There are, according to Humphrey, two deaths: the still, safe, balance of the vertical static death (the Apollonian) and the wild, exciting, dynamic death of the off-balance (the Dionysian). For Humphrey all movement takes place between these two extremes, and she referred to this as 'the arc between two deaths'. Between these two points there is the rebound from fall (Dionysian) to recovery (Apollonian). This sequence — fall, rebound, recovery — echoes the human instincts which come into play when we fall, and was based on Humphrey's study of natural movement patterns. Emotionally and thematically in Humphrey's dances, the principle represents the excitement or fear of the fall and the repose or peace of recovery. Her style, which is based on simple movements like running, breathing, standing, leaping, rising, is characterized by action and reaction, yielding to gravity and resistance to gravity, force countered yb force. It is a lyrical style expressive of the innate power of the human spirit to triumph over adverse forces.

José Limon was a student, fellow dancer and collaborator of Doris Humphrey. Supported in his decision to form his own company, in 1945 (Humphrey choreographed for him) Limon developed the Humphrey technique into his own particular style through choreographic exploration. He also devised a series of exercises to isolate the various parts of the body in order that students should learn to control the weight and functioning of each with an aim to achieve the fluid, harmonious working of the whole body as a single unit. These exercises were based on his concept of the body as an orchestra, and the process of learning to dance as one of learning to play each of the instruments separately, then together. But his contribution to the technique was also as a great artist. A romantic, impulsive man, handsome in the heroic mould, one of his great contributions to modern dance was to create an expression for male passion and strength and to develop male roles in richness and status. This was an inspiration to scores of future male dancers, and continues to attract men to the Limon technique.

The Humphrey/Limon technique demands physical strength and lays emphasis on using the whole body as an expressive tool. The dramatic and emotional charge is high – 'The struggle of muscles is a metaphor for the struggle of souls', a critic once commented. In his teaching Limon put emphasis on hard work, sweat and guts, and for his choreography he chose heroic, universal themes based on religious and historical subjects.

Merce Cunningham, like José Limon, belongs to the second generation of modern dance. From 1940–45 Cunningham was a member of the Martha Graham Company and, despite his subsequent rejection of her precepts, his dance still retains some of the nervous tension and implosive impact of the Graham style. Cunningham has come to be seen as a figurehead of the second generation of modern dance, and as the father of the post-moderns, in his rejection of dance as an expression of the human condition and his focus on the presentation of movement for its own sake. He believes that dance should be easeful on the body not stressful (the crux of his rejection of Graham), and he was the first to incorporate everyday movements into dance.

The Merce Cunningham Dance Company was established in 1953. Cunningham's long association with the contemporary composer, John Cage, led him to formulate a new aesthetic: dance is dance, music is music, and neither need to be dependent on the other. Cunningham technique is based on the kinetic integrity of the body, the intrinsic movement and phrasing which stems from the body's internal rhythm, unconstrained by the melodic or formal proposals of external music. He also maintains that dance need not be based on philosophical or psychological material. Dance for its own sake speaks for itself. Although inevitably connotations will always be evoked in the imagination of the spectators.

Early on Cunningham introduced chance into his choreography. Sometimes he threw pennies or cast the I Ching to determine the steps of the dancers or the length of a piece. He initiated the concept of 'open form' in which various secions or elements of a piece could be played in a number of different sequences or combinations.

Cunningham is unique in our time in having gathered together over the years a distinguished collection of composers, musicians, painters and designers for his performances. Only the great ballet impresario Diaghilev had achieved such a conglomeration of talent.

To watch, the Cunningham style is magnetic but unflashy. The dance is not built around one dancer or an obvious tour de force, climax, or splendid virtuosity. Silence and stillness play vital parts in his choreography. The precision, skill and abstract power are indisputable and exciting to watch and, for the dancer, challenging to master.

For the non-professional, the Cunningham technique offers a rigorous and exacting training. Having taken the ballet barre and placed it, as it were, in the middle of the studio, the dancer is forced to develop a strong centre, internal balance and alignment.

In class you would learn elements of ballet footwork, and isolation in different areas of the torso and back along the lines of modern dance principles. Emphasis is on using the torso as freely as possible on top of complex leg work. There is an austerity and discipline in Cunningham that will appeal to those with a taste for contemporary art and music, for the abstractions of pure maths, computers, electronics or the clear inner spaces of meditation and Zen.

In her book on modern dance, the American writer and dance critic Margaret Lloyd sums up the departure that modern dance took from classical ballet:

Modern dance is a matter of dynamic volume rather than of presentation solely on the frontal plane, of mass more than of line. Being more concerned with the abstraction of things felt than with the pictorial representation of things seen, it chooses broken rhythms, off-balances, the casual appearance, the imperfect cadence, in preference to what is smooth and formal and regular.

Modern dance techniques have much to offer us. They are all of them demanding physically and technically, requiring dedication and regular work to produce satisfying results – so they will not appeal to the casual exerciser concerned solely with keeping the body in trim. However to the person seeking a richer meaning to movement these styles are ideal. They do not demand such set body types as ballet but they are as equally demanding in terms of mastering the exercises and technique. One major advantage is that you can start training in modern dance at a much later age without prejudicing either your development or the pleasure you derive.

What these styles have to offer in particular is the richness of dramatic and emotional expression. This is where theatre and dance meet most profoundly. While there is certainly joy and exuberance to be found here, modern dance is essentially very serious in its concerns. Those who feel themselves to be involved in the whys, wherefores and hows of the human condition will find much to sympathise with in these forms.

The satisfaction derived from understanding and developing the expressive power of the body goes beyond the experience of simply moving well for its own sake. These methdos will appeal to all those who feel a need for this extra dimension and who want creatively to combine the joy of movement with rigorous technique and dramatic expression.

Dance techniques come in and out of fashion so you may have to search a bit to find a pure Graham, Humphrey or Cunningham class. However, many teachers trained in these techniques incorporate them inot more general modern dance classes. The growing interest in dance will hopefully encourage more classes teaching the original techniques.

Post-Modern Dance

In the 1960s conceptualism hit the arts. The visual arts, music and contemporary dance became more interested in exploring and developing ideas, theories and systems than in expressing emotions or providing a pleasurable experience for the spectator. Coupled with this was the desire of many dancers to remove dance from its romantic pedestal and make it more accessible to the ordinary person, more in touch with 'real life'. So over the following decades, dancers experimented with abolishing costume and sets, with incorporating task movements (e.g. sweeping the floor) and simple daily movements (e.g.

walking). They tried unusual venues (to get dance out of the theatre and, sometimes literally, on to the streets) and encouraged audience participation. This new era was dubbed the Post-modern.

Contact improvisation was created by Steve Paxton, an American dancer who trained with Merce Cunningham and then became involved with the dance experimentation taking place in the 1960s and 70s in New York. Contact is a duet dance form: an approach to dance which involves partners moving in physical contact and mutually exploring the pathways which develop between them. The aim of Contact is not to present a uniform style (as in classical or modern dance), but the specific techniques do create a recognizable form.

Paxton studied t'ai-chi, yoga and especially aikido for many years and Contact owes a lot to the principles of this martial art. 'They are both partnering forms and both are concerned with a very light and appropriate use of energy in fairly dangerous situations, one an act of aggression, the other an act of dance', said Paxton in an interview conducted at Dartington College in 1981. Both forms use spherical movements and the idea of extension – that is, of feeling *through* the thing you touch, so that, just as for example, a blind man can feel the quality of the ground through his cane as an extension of his arms, so the dancer or aikidoist should be able to feel the other's energy and beyond that the gravity and support of the ground.

Both forms stress the need to be in touch with your centre. But while aikido is potentially about a life or death situation, Contact is the reverse:

> Instead of keeping your centre away from somebody else as the martial arts do, instead of fending them off, you are allowing them into your centre . . . or to depend physically upon your balance, your centre of mass for their own movement. And you're doing the same with them. You are mutually employing each other's leverage.

The two elements most emphasized in Contact are *focus* and *peripheral sense*, allowing hearing and feeling to come into play. Just as it emphasizes using all the senses, so Contact emphasizes using the whole body. In fact in early lessons students are asked not to use their hands at all in order to get away from habit. So the student learns to use the upper arm the thigh, the torso. In this the student is also learning to manipulate the heavier weights of the body in a more refined way.

Whereas in ballet or modern dance you focus on a specific isolated body part, like the foot, pelvis or arm, in Contact you stay aware of the whole body as well as being aware of the situation and the movements around you.

Contact involves support and trust and much of the class deals with developing this between participants and in the individual. The body has powerful inbuilt reflexes to avoid hurting itself, and learning to trust these automatic reflexes is another part of Contact. This psychological element can have an emotionally therapeutic effect and develop great kinaesthetic sensitivity. The form involves much energetic work – lifts, falls, whirling movements, often at great speed – as well as the slower, more sensitive explorations of Contact..

There is a very pragmatic feeling to Contact. It is not dramatic, nor emotional and certainly not mystical. Students are reminded to keep their eyes open and the intimate physical contact is never seen as sexual or aggressive – a neutral approach is the one Paxton recommends. The dance is, on one level, about processing physical information – skin touching skin, the difference between air and mass, the feel and knowledge of joints, muscles, bones; and, on another level, it is about building up a finely tuned awareness of the inner and the outer.

Contact Improvisation is very suited to beginners because it requires no previous training and there is no emphasis on skill or technique. It attracts far more men than most dance forms. Perhaps because the form is very hard work, with as much emphasis on acrobatic work as on the quieter, slower movements.

There is little emphasis on performance in Britain although the situation is somewhat different in the United States where there is also a magazine, *Contact Quarterly*, which provides a forum for new ideas in this ever developing form.

Release Work is a broad term to describe the different work being done by dance teachers in this field. There is no one method but behind all the varying approaches lies the work of Mabel Ellsworth Todd, an American who devoted her life to the study and teaching of what she called 'bodily economy'. She combined the study of physics, mechanics, anatomy and physiology to provide, in a seminal book called *The Thinking Body*, published in 1937, a full and detailed account of the way the body moves and functions in action. Todd deals with the habits of movement we build up, with the psycho-physical mechanisms involved in resisting gravity (one of the major sources of postural problems), with the saving of energy in movement, with breathing, and with relaxation – 'the crying need of our age', which she already recognized in the mid 1930s.

Release work has as its precept the releasing of habitual blocks and patterns of movement to enable the most efficient use of the body. In this, Release is similar to therapeutic movement forms. However the approach is quite different due to the fact that it has been developed by dancers, such as Mary Fulerson, working at Dartington College, in Devon, and Joan Skinner and Marsha Paludan in the United States. Creative dance rather than therapy is their focus.

A central concept that Release work shares with the Alexander Technique is that the bones not the muscles should support the body, and emphasis is placed on the vertebral axis of the spine. Breathing is focused upon as providing a fundamental body rhythm and information about the interior of the body. Breath is seen as the continuous thread through all the movement. Students become aware of the direction of body energy and learn to listen to their body through very simple actions, such as curling and uncurling, sitting, crawling, squatting, standing, walking, running, jumping, falling, turning. Many of these movements deliberately recall the developmental movement patterns of the body that a baby goes through from the foetal stage up to adult stances.

Fulkerson emphasizes developing the quality of patience and the positive attributes of stillness. And much of the work is done through imagery. Students work with the shapes the body makes – the 'bowls' of the pelvis and shoulder girdle, the spheres the body can create in movement, and also with imaginative, poetic images given to them by the teacher or produced by themselves.

Listening to the body is important. Most of the time we tell our bodies what to do, but rarely, except in response to urgent needs like hunger, do we allow our bodies to direct the action.

Release work stimulates personal movement exploration and develops a heightened capacity to listen and respond to the language of the imagination. This work is rich resource for all those doing creative work and a good training for the performer.

Fulkerson defines technique as 'the integration of idea and acts and it is the result of the persistent dialogue between demand and patience.' Relations of space and time are principal concerns and in a sense release involves going back to basics: getting to feel the support of the ground, yielding to its support to enable you to spring up and off into action. Eastern principles of yin and yang also lie behind these concepts. While for some the work may be too soft and slow, for others the increased awareness of the deeper muscles and functioning of the dynamic body and the sense of a flowing line (rather than isolated body parts) is exhilarating and rewarding.

Release work, as its generalized title suggests, is not a definitive school, but a growing, changing approach made up of a number of individual teachers. Working with this kind of dance has a great deal to offer to those who want to cultivate their intuitive side, their kinaesthetic sense and awareness of their body in relation to themselves and others, and who prefer the expressive, dynamic movements of dance to the more regulated exercises of movement re-education techniques.

The avenues opened up by the innovators of the 1960s and 70s have proved valuable, not only in terms of injecting new vitality into dance performance but also, by de-emphasizing technique and virtuosity, in providing a rich world of possibility for the non-professional who wishes to dance for pleasure.

The Chantraine Method

This is one of the most inclusive methods of dance available today and as such ideally suited to the non-professional who would like to get fit while exploring the creative aspects of dance as fully as possible.

The method was created in France by Françoise and Alain Chantraine in the late 1950s. After a rich and varied career in the arts (as musicians and teachers of dance) and studies in psychology and kinesiology, their search was for a method of teaching dance which would use the whole person – the mental, emotional and physical – and which would integrate dance with life so that they became not different in kind but only in degree. The school they created has as its aim 'movement and dance as aids to the development of the person'. And from this the traditional emphasis on performance in dance gave way in importance to emphasis on the life and experience of the person dancing.

Three basic principles underlie the Chantraine method and put the founders' research into practical form. The first is the notion of different energy states. Students become familiar with these, learn to use energy in an appropriate way, so increasing their energy potential. In this way passivity, moving into 'neutral', and learning to use stillness are just as important as being able to use maximum energy and move at high speed – as well as all the stages in between.

The second principle is based on the idea of the 'five times of life'. These are: rhythm, interiority, construction, forms and choreography. Every class is structured so as to give a period of time to each of these concepts, to alternate between them and learn to combine them.

Rhythm deals with personal tempo, with the ability to refine and vary one's range of speeds, and with rhythm in space: height, depth and breadth, and with exploring the different sensations of weight during locomotion. It includes an 'endurance' section, in which energy is used to the maximum.

Interiority concerns the opposite to rhythm, that of going inwards and becoming passive. The student learns to relax completely on the floor and become conscious of inner processes and of the infinities of time and space. After an initial stillness this follows a certain pattern of movements which explore growth. The students do these exercises moving from a lying position with their eyes closed, each individual doing the same movements but at her own pace, like a slow group dance out of sync.

In construction, the student learns how to master place and function. There are two aspects which are important and em-phasized in the teaching of construction: the development of a well-centred energy core and a well-held spine and pelvis (see Posture pages 128–138).

The last two 'times' aim to bring the individual into contact and collaboration with the other members of the group. Form is concerned with expression, so the student develops a range of expressive dance forms: curves, volumes, straight lines, angles, forms deriving from art, architecture and nature. The emphasis is on creativity both alone and in dialogue with other members of the class. Choreography is just that: the coming together of the whole class to work on a choreographed piece of work. It is also the 'time' for dance as an art, when all the other 'times' come together to create an integrated work.

The third principle underlying the Chantraine Method is a psychological approach. Rather than focus on a notion of striving or hard work in order to get somewhere, students are encouraged to look for the things they like in an exercise, to look for the positive way forward and act upon this. To this end a class will have plenty of opportunity for discussion and sharing of the experience of an exercise, of how to proceed with a choreography, of what they would like to concentrate on next, and so on.

Chantraine is a method but not a single style: it is eclectic in its use of techniques. Exercises might derive from classical ballet, from Graham, jazz, even newer techniques, as well as from re-education methods such as yoga, or Feldenkrais, all according to the needs and ages of the pupils and the orientation of a particular class. The richness of influence, in both technique and music is marked in the the choreographies too: pieces may range from an angular rhythmic piece danced to Bach, to a jazzy, syncopated number to music by Diana Ross.

Chantraine is a method suitable and adaptable to all ages, from three years old to 80, and to all levels of ability. Teachers often work with psychologists and psychomotricians and also give demonstrations of the technique with their pupils at a variety of events throughout the year.

Martial Arts

These days one is just as likely to see someone practising t'ai chi ch'uan forms in the park of an early morning as going for a run or doing calisthenics. Yet this invasion by the Eastern martial arts began only in the last century and made almost no ingress in Europe and America until after the Second World War when returning soldiers began to practise and pass on some of the skills they had picked up from the masters in Japan and Korea. But the martial arts were truly popularized in the West most dramatically through the remarkable films of Kurosawa in the 1950s, such as *The Seven Samurai*, and then in the 1970s by the legendary Bruce Lee, whose extraordinary skills converted millions overnight to the ferocious beauty of the Eastern martial arts.

Today we think of martial arts as being exclusively from the East, but the West also has its martial tradition. The word comes from Mars, the Greek god of war. War is not the prerogative of China and Japan! Plato wrote of fighting without an antagonist (shadow boxing); military dances, boxing and wrestling were all part of Greek combat training, and wrestling featured in the first Olympic games. Archery, jousting and mock battles were the Wimbledons and Ascots of the middle ages, and long before the likes of Mohammed Ali or Barry McGuigan, boxing was a widespread sport in the West.

While in the West martial practices have long been superceded by sports and athletics in mass popularity, they have endured so powerfully in the East because of the philosophy and approach that lie behind them, making them more a way of life than merely effective combat techniques.

The martial arts were preceded by a long military tradition in China. Extended periods of fierce warfare among the kingdoms bred some brilliant strategists and generals, the most famous of which was Sun Tzu, whose book *The Art of War* (written about 350 BC) is still required reading in China and was read devotedly by Mao Tse-Tung. But it was around the same period that the seeds of change were being sown and two individuals were to profoundly influence not only martial practices but the whole religious thought and practice of the East.

The philosophies that underpin all the martial arts are Taoism and Buddhism. The first was developed by the great spiritual teacher Lao Tzu in China around 300 BC, and the second was brought to China in the early 6th century BC by a Buddhist monk called Bodidharma who settled in the Shaolin Temple at the foot of the Songshan mountains. It was here and through the teachings of Bodidharma (called Ta Mo by the Chinese) that the existing Chinese martial practices were codified and infused with the meditative and spiritual depths which transformed them into arts. From here originated the tradition known as Shaolin boxing.

It was at the Shaolin Temple, that the meditative practices of Buddhism were amalgamated with the breathing, energizing, pragmatic approach of Taoism and combined with the combat skills already being taught (even monks had to protect themselves from attack in such remote areas). This marriage of Buddhism with Taoism expressed in movement and fighting forms created a belief system of spiritual practices and martial arts which offered such a universal, cohesive and powerful approach to living that it remains central to life in the East to this day. In practising martial arts one is able to experience and embody the very principles and beliefs which lie at the core of Eastern civilisation and give meaning to the very existence of its peoples. 'Meditation in activity is a hundred, a thousand, a million times superior to meditation in repose', said a Chinese ancient.

Bodidharma brought to the martial pratices the concept of *wou-te* (martial virtue or discipline) – humility, restraint, discipline and respect for human life. While his principal concern was the propagation of the Buddhist texts, Bodidharma taught his disciples breathing and exercise techniques to alleviate the mental and physical strain of the many hours of meditation and reading the monks underwent as part of their studies. In this way he instilled the idea of practising martial arts not for fighting but for strengthening the body and maintaining health.

Thus the Shaolin tradition focused on healing; the emphasis is on balancing the various forces in the body. Equilibrium remains a key concept in the martial arts as it does in certain healing arts, like acupuncture, expressed by such theories as the energy meridians, and the five element theory (earth, water, wood, fire and metal).

Prior to Bodidharma's codification and expansion Chinese martial artists trained primarily to fight, and it is recounted that they were fond of bullying the weak. The concept of *wu-te* brought about a change in this misuse of power and promoted the idea of spiritual development through the martial arts.

Martial virtue finds its ultimate expression many centuries later in the Japanese concept of *Bushido* – Way of the Warrior. The warrior class, called samurai, developed a tremendous system of moral codes which embodied laws on right and wrong in every area of life and bound them tightly to their families, clans and their place in the social structure. While martial arts disciplines were already widely practised in Japan by the eleventh and twelfth centuries, the idea of Bushido was not fully codified until the seventeenth century.

In Japan the martial arts developed in conjunction with Zen Buddhism, a religion which is Taoist in character. Pragmatic, to do with the way (*tao*) you live life rather than with metaphysics, the virtues which characterize *Bushido* reflect this: justice, courage, benevolence, politeness, veracity, honour and loyalty. All martial arts in Japan were initially called bujutsu (*bu*=martial, *jutsu*=skill/art), but during the long, peaceful Edo period (1603–1867) since combat training was in less demand, martial arts came to be transformed into a spiritual path, to be referred to as *Budo* (*bu*=martial, *do*=way, from the Chinese *tao*).

In Japan today both the *Budo* system and an earlier system, known as *Bugei*, are taught. The distinction is an important one. The two systems run parallel, so that the combative *Bugei* forms like kenjutsu, iajutsu, jujutsu are mirrored by the stylized *Budo* forms, kendo, iaido and judo, which emphasize the mental, physical and spiritual development of the individual not just the fighting skill.

In Japan the martial arts are quite formalized and uniform in the basic skills and applications, and training usually conforms to an agreed system. In China, however, there are literally hundreds of different forms and systems, stemming from the establishment in the seventeenth century of the Ch'ing Dynasty. Fearing an uprising of trained fighters against the new regime, the martial arts were discouraged and went underground, with one teacher passing on his knowledge in secret to a select few of his family or close friends. The heritage of a particular form became like a family tree and so present day teachers talk of being the direct inheritor of this or that master's tradition. While based on the same training principle of repetition until moves become reflexive, all have different training routines, different techniques and emphases.

The principal division that can be made in this huge diversity of styles and techniques in China is between the internal and the external systems, sometimes described as the soft and hard schools. The systems refer more to a basic approach than to any fixed categorization since many of the forms use ideas from both systems.

The internal system (exemplified by t'ai chi) derives ultimately from the teachings of Lao Tzu whose Tao Te Ching (The Way and the Power) penetrates beneath the hard and fixed world, where it would appear that the strong conquers the weak, and uncovers the hidden laws of nature:

> Nothing in the heaven is softer or more yielding than water; but when it attacks things hard and resistant there is not one of them that can prevail. For they can find no way of altering it. That the yielding conquers the resistant and soft conquers the hard is a fact known by all men, yet utilised by none.

Taoist doctrine talks of *wu wei* (non action) and *tzu jan* (spontaneous or natural) which in martial arts terms characterize the internal systems by the principle of refraining from contention, finding a way to move through the world, or work with your partner, in harmony and balance with the forces around you. Actions should be spontaneous and effortless and adapted to the circumstances of each new situation. The focus is on vital energy (*chi*), will and internal strength, with an emphasis on using minimal effort, thereby conserving your vital energy in action. The internal systems, aim to train the mind in order to outwit opponents rather than using muscular strength. The force used is centred, flowing outwards and merging with the opponent's force to unbalance him with his own power. Breathing practices emphasize this: the practitioner learns to breathe low into the abdomen, or centre of gravity, some two inches below the navel, the point known in Chinese as *tan-tien* (*hara* in Japanese) which is the respository of chi. Such abdominal breathing helps ground the individual and draw energy up from the earth as well. Hsing I and pa-kua in China, aikido and judo in Japan are developments of the internal, soft approach.

The external system (exemplified by kung fu) is linked more strongly with the Shaolin Temple practices. The fundamental principle is that force can be opposed with force. Practices involve striking blows with hands, fists, elbow, feet, knees and head. The emphasis is on attack, and counter attacks are met with blocks which become re-attack and so on. Since blows are most effective when delivered in a straight line, much training focuses on lining up the body behind the attack so as to use the whole body energy most efficiently. Development of physical strength, principally muscular power, is a central aim since the fighting style of the external forms is primarily a contest of strength combined with skill and speed. Breathing is focused at a point between the solar plexus and the upper chest. The abdomen is not fully expanded so that a high pressure can be created in the chest allowing for an explosive burst of energy and concentrated power. Controlling this energy and not expending it too quickly is very important in the hard martial art forms. Karate in Japan, tae kwon do in Korea and Thai boxing in Thailand all developed from this hard approach.

The interplay of the two systems is shown in this passage from the teachings of a contemporary master of the arts, Hung I-hsiang:

Strength always moves in one direction. A curve and a straight line meet at only one point. To attack one must strive to push one's strength against this point from the most advantageous angle. To defend, one must strive to avoid the point of contact. The most vital skill in this process is to learn how to find the point and the proper angle for maximum thrust, and then apply full strength to it at the moment of contact.

Most people believe that the shortest distance between two points is a straight line. Therefore, direct frontal attacks are usually swift and ferocious. Consequently, most martial arts techniques emphasize circling. The main idea is to avoid direct confrontation between two direct lines because this is self-defeating. Since there is a limit to an opponent's speed it is always possible to deflect a direct frontal attack by employing a suitable angle. There is a motto in martial arts that says: 'Emphasize the inner meaning, not the outer strength.' If I find you to be more powerful than me, I will never take a blow from you, for that would be useless. If I am more powerful, however, I will not let you go. (Howard Reid and Michael Crowther, *The Way of the Warrior*, Century 1983.)

As the Shaolin tradition developed in China, different approaches to the martial arts formed in the north and south of the country, styles which reflect, it is said, the differences in terrain. The hills and rolling plains of the north, and the practice of horse-riding contributed to strong legs, essential in the kicks and jumps so typical of the northern school of martial arts. In the south the extensive system of waterways developed the upper body through rowing and poling, and this is reflected in the many hand and fist striking techniques, and the emphasis on steady, rooted balance (to earth or boat) typical of the southern school.

There are two other important aspects of the martial arts which offer something very valuable to the practitioner, amateur or otherwise, not found in most Western sports and movement forms. The first is the opportunity to come to grips with violence and aggression. These are facts of life both within individual nature and in the world around us. In fact such has been the rise in muggings, harassment and attack in the streets of cities, that more and more people are turning to martial arts and self-defence courses based on martial techniques, simply to protect themselves. But the martial arts offer more than a good defence technique. They allow us to explore, experience and to some degree sublimate the violent feelings inside us, our 'shadow' side, within the bounds of accepted social behaviour. Through this we can come to understand these impulses better, develop a relationship with what is seen as the 'negative' aspect of ourselves and so find ways of using that energy creatively rather than, as is usually the case, self-destructively.

The second aspect of the martial arts so valuable to us is the incorporation of a deep and ancient spiritual tradition within a movement form. Rather than having to go to a special place, like a church, to withdraw from the world and the 'evils of the flesh', to abstain and chastise, which are the routes to spiritual experience via the traditional religions of the West and East, the practitioner of martial arts can experience the integration of Self, the sense of stillness and centredness in activity itself. No other movement forms offer this so completely. In a sense, they help return us to the original significance of the earliest Olympian games when the martial skills of that earlier epoch were practised as a part of a religious festival and as a re-dedication of the body, emotions and mind of the individual to his soul and his commitment to God in whatever form the deity was experienced by him. If physical training and a martial arts regime can help recapture that connection with our inner self, and with a greater whole beyond our individual needs, then there is every reason to understand their widespread and dramatic growth in the last few decades.

T'ai-Chi Ch'uan

T'ai-chi ch'uan, or as it is more often called, t'ai-chi, is practised by more people than any other form of martial art. In China it is practised by millions of people every day and in the morning mists it is commonplace to see groups and individuals in town squares and parks quietly going through their forms. T'ai-chi ch'uan is the most common of the schools which derive from the internal or soft system of the Shaolin tradition of martial arts. As such it involves a more inward focused attention and emphasis is less on sinew and bones as on internal sensation, feeling and energy. Of all the systems, it most clearly reflects its Taoist heritage in its practice and its philosophy. T'ai-chi ch'uan translates into The Supreme Pole Fist.

At first appearance it could easily be mistaken for a dance or gentle ballet, so hidden are the martial arts components of the forms. Movement is gentle and easy, little force or effort seems to be exerted. Students are asked to follow the lead of the teacher as one movement flows into the next. But all of the different movements can be translated into actual martial arts attacks or defensive manoeuvres.

There are five principles which govern the physical use of the body. *First*, the movements are performed in as relaxed and comfortable a position as possible. The whole torso is gentle and supple, with body weight settling to the floor and feet. To help with attaining this relaxed posture the movements are always done slowly and gently.

Secondly gentle breathing through the nose and using the diaphragm rather than the ribs and intercostal muscles is emphasized.

Thirdly the waist must be flexible as it is the focus of most movements. Arm and hand movements must be incorporated into the movement of the waist. This of course emphasizes the importance of posture and alignment. Since all large body movements originate in the pelvis and waist it also follows that even small and gentle movements should have a pelvic component.

The *fourth* principle is more subtle but even more concerned with posture and alignment. The sacrum should be held vertically or tipped down to facilitate the *chi* (energy) reaching the top of the head so that the head is held as if gently floating or almost suspended from above. The body is held in a way 'so light that the addition of a feather will be felt, and so pliable that a fly cannot alight on it without setting it in motion.' (Drager)

The *fifth* principle stresses that all movements have a circular component. Since force opposed by force will result in the stronger force prevailing, all t'ai-chi ch'uan movements focus on re-directing the opposing force and neutralizing it through circular movements.

A great deal of time in t'ai-chi ch'uan is spent in the slow practice of the forms. Different schools and teachers will have different forms but they are all practiced slowly, gently and in coordination with all the members of a class. The other two major training practices are called, 'pushing hands' and 'sticking hands'. In pushing hands partners take turns directing a straight line push towards the other which is fended off by a number of circular movements which are part of the forms practised. While in the West this is rhythmic and almost ritualized, in the East it is quite vigorous and energetic. In the other exercise, sticking hands, one individual puts his hand on top of his partner's and then the partner moves his hands in a variety of ways. The aim is to keep your hand on top of your partner's throughout the movement.

T'ai-chi training usually starts with considerable time spent doing solo movement: practising the form. Subsequently one will move on to pushing hands and sticking hands. Eventually, after some years and if your teacher is inclined in that direction, some practising of free fighting may be allowed. Self-defence is considered the final stage in development as the defensive nature of the system is emphasized in line with the basic non-violent attitude of Taoism.

There are two other major forms of internal system martial arts: hsing-i and pa-kua. Hsing-i is often taught as a preliminary martial art to t'ai-chi ch'uan. It focuses more on vertical strength and at times almost linear movements. It is similar in appearance to the harder forms of Shaolin boxing and still operates on the principle of strength to oppose strength. But the practitioner keeps low to the floor, sometimes almost crouching and the defensive movements are more rounded. In addition it is permeated with the Taoist principles of the softer arts. Hsing-i translates as *hsing* (form) and *i* as (intention or idea). A master at hsing-i should be able to read the intention of the opponent's form and avoid an advance, or anticipate and counter without difficulty.

The second major form is known as pa-kua. This is sometimes taught as a follow-on from the hsing-i form. In pa-kua the emphasis is on constant change and unpredictable movements. Whereas hsing-i is more straight and linear, pa-kua is all curves and circles. It is more evasive than hsing-i and is based upon the eight trigrams of the I Ching, the ancient Chinese oracle, used to predict possible choices of action. The philosophy of I Ching is a very central belief system based upon the interaction of the polar forces of Yin and Yang. In embodying the I Ching, pa-kua emphasizes constantly changing patterns and possible variations. The emphasis is on evasion and concealment so that sometimes the martial component is not easily recognized in pa-kua. The emphasis is on horizontal strength. The hands are more open than hsing-i, and the movements have a circular dance-like fluidity.

T'ai-chi is the epitome of the soft form of the martial arts. It is the one martial art which works most directly with relaxation and stress reduction during the actual practise of the form. The speed and pace of the practice allows one to lower the arousal level to the point where things like the startle reflex and the fight or flight reflex can actually be interrupted through training in self-defence. Consequently, t'ai-chi is perhaps the best martial art for the cultivation of posture and alignment. The central position with legs slightly bent, pelvis dropped under the lumbar region of the spine, the narrow vertical central axis, the circular movements around the centre axis, the gentle but full range of movement of the arms and legs all result in a constant re-alignment of the entire body around the spine with a resultant small moment of inertia (see page 133).

Strength *per se* is not emphasized and it is possible to practice t'ai-chi without concerning yourself with how strong you must become. The power of the system as a form of self-defence derives from the focus on neuromuscular coordination and a constant refinement of the subtle skills acquired through the practice of the form. In addition, the emphasis on cultivating *tan-tien* or *hara*, that central point of balance and energy below the navel, helps create an atmosphere in a t'ai-chi class which often resembles a movement awareness class like Feldenkrais or Eutony. Awareness is a central quality to most t'ai-chi classes.

Of all the martial arts, t'ai-chi ch'uan is the least martial in form. This makes it a welcome form for women, older people or anyone who wants to feel the benefits of a martial arts tradition whilst avoiding the more aggressive aspects of some of the other arts. T'ai-chi places emphasis on self-mastery and also on unity. It speaks most directly to those who are looking for the spiritual or transcendent element since this is an overt objective for t'ai-chi practitioners.

Kung Fu

Kung fu originally meant 'the practice of martial arts exercises', so all martial arts could be said to involve kung fu. But the name is now generally used to include a number of the external or hard systems of the martial arts which are descended from the Chinese Shaolin Temple tradition. There are about 400 different major styles which are grouped under kung fu including ones with names like white crane, horse, praying mantis, etc.

One distinction which can be made within the kung fu or

Shaolin external systems is between the northern and southern styles, reflecting, it is said, the differences in terrain.

The northern approach embodies a style of athleticism and grace, of the dramatic leaps of the Peking Opera and the explosive speed of kung fu. Stances are wide, arms and legs fully extended in attack; emphasis is placed on explosive attacks and sweeping movements. As spectacular as the high flying kicks are, many martial artists question the extravagance of these techniques, except for special circumstances – unseating a rider from a horse, for instance (hardly an everyday occurrence). They leave the attacker open to counter attack, and it is hard to alter the trajectory, or the attack itself, in mid flight. It is easy to be unbalanced but one advantage is the element of surprise the northern style offers.

The southern school is quite different. Practitioners maintain a solid, grounded stance which leads to extensive development of shoulders and arms. Sudden overpowering movements, named after the animals they resemble (tiger, leopard, eagle and monkey for instance) are performed with great force, and the emphasis is on simultaneous attack and defence. Very quick, reflexive actions are cultivated which produce the effect of continuous motion, a shower of blows and blocks, giving the opponent nothing to get hold of.

The oldest kung fu traditions were derived from various approaches characterized by five animals representing different forms in relationship to hard and soft or internal and external. The dragon was the first form and focuses on the development of *shen* which is roughly translated as spirit or mind. It is the gentlest of the Shaolin animal forms and though not practised in its original form anymore probably is closest to t'ai-chi.

The snake form focuses on chi and its movements are coiling and circling like a snake. They appear soft and flowing but there is an emphasis on inner strength like that of a coiled snake ready to strike. It resembles the internal martial art pa-kua.

The tiger form is again characterized by its name. Emphasis is placed on the bones and power. Movements are extremely energetic and furious and there is a sense of overwhelming the opponent.

The fourth form, the leopard, is like the tiger in generating powerful movements and attacks but there is more grace, and the sudden leaps resemble a sinewy leopard.

The last animal form, the crane, is evocative of the angular movements of a bird. There are in and out movements like pecking and blocking techniques which look wing-like. The emphasis is on the sinews and there is also a focus on balance like a tall crane. Posture and alignment are important.

There are other forms of kung fu which use animal names like the monkey, the praying mantis, the white crane, which all evoke the animal after which they are named.

Whatever style you pursue, kung fu, or Shaolin external systems of boxing, involve the development of physical strength. In some schools, as well as practicing the forms, time is spent on strength training, But these forms also require very quick reflexive responses. Bruce Lee, the most famous of kung fu practitioners (probably the most famous of all contemporary martial artists in the public eye), was well known for his demonstration of speed and agility. Lee would stand 8 feet away from a karate black belt informing him where he was going to attack and with which hand. Still Lee could cross the distance and deliver the blow before the opponent could adopt a defensive block.

Breathing techniques are emphasized but the focus is placed between the solar plexus and chest. This produces a more powerful generation of energy and, as a result, a more explosive blow than the softer forms of Shaolin. However, amongst many experts this form of breathing is considered to be dangerous. In fact, while Bruce Lee is said to have died of a cerebral haemorrhage, many martial arts masters have suggested that his death may have been in part due to the misuse of certain breath-holding *chi*-generating exercises involving the chest and solar plexus. In the long run it is important to develop deeper levels of breathing which draw their power from the *hara* or *tan-tien*. It takes longer to develop and the results tend to be more sustained rather than explosive, but they stand you in better stead for building an effective technique and for general health and well being.

Like all martial arts, the cultivation of kung fu techniques results in a definite sense of self-mastery. Centring is important, but some kung fu systems do not devote very much attention to spiritual practices. There is less emphasis on *hara* and *tan-tien* cultivating techniques. Because of the wide range of schools and teachers and no central agreement as to what constitutes kung fu, do investigate the history of the school and teacher you choose to follow. Be discriminating.

Judo

Judo was probably the first martial art which came to be known outside the East amongst a wide number of people. It was brought back from Japan by American and European soldiers after the end of the Second World War. It is undoubtedly the most popular martial art form in Japan with over eight million people practising it regularly. There is some confusion about the name because some people say they practice jujitsu or jujutsu as opposed to judo. Jujutsu is the antecedent of judo. It covers a range of 700 officially documented systems which developed in the sixteenth and seventeenth centuries in Japan after the Shogunate brought all of the warring clans under its umbrella and it was no longer necessary to have so many combative samurai. It should be stressed that while jujutsu designates primarily any empty-handed system, it was meant to operate as a complementary martial art to the use of weapons, particularly the sword. In other words, when close combat required hand-to-hand combat, then it took over where weapons left off although some forms of jujutsu include small hand weapons. It is because of this use that jujutsu developed into a grappling, throwing, close quarters system of techniques. Jujutsu means the Art of Flexibility, and employs a wide range of techniques from grappling and throwing to striking, kicking and arm-locking as well as strangleholds and *atemi* (attacking weak points).

In the last half of the nineteenth century a man named Kano Jigori studied the variety of jujutsu systems and began to formalize an approach to them which included not only the physical and moral systems of the Jujutsu tradition but also the increased use of the martial art for physical training and education, in recognition of the need to eliminate some of the more lethal aspects of the system. He also wanted to develop a system of training which could be incorporated into the educational system of Japan. Ju-do or the Way of Flexibility, was the result.

One of the central principles behind judo is the notion of

using the opponent's own force to defeat him. So following on from the t'ai chi ch'uan and pa-kua approaches, the opponent's energy is redirected in a way to throw him off balance and defeat him. Kano developed a regime of techniques and eventually his system became known as Kodokan, or 'the place of the path of creation'. Judo is essentially a grappling art. Contestants tend to stand at close quarters holding on to each other's jackets or arms, and manoeuvering to gain a position in which the opponent's own strength can be used to throw him. Footwork is very important in training. Having thrown an opponent, the object is then to pin him, hold him with a joint lock, or subdue him with a stranglehold. In judo competitions in Japan, the stranglehold can be applied and often is to the point where the opponent loses consciousness. Most properly qualified teachers of judo are also taught resuscitation techniques! This extreme is not usually practiced in Western schools and certainly not in beginners' classes!

Kano stressed two principles: one he called 'the principle of right use of energy'. This refers to the use of the opponent's own energy against himself and the constant maintenance of one's centre without being thrown off balance. The other principle is: 'The principle of mutual welfare'. In classes, much of the training centres around free-form grappling with a succession of opponents during a class period. Opponents are faced and met one after another until the individuals are exhausted. Because of this it is important to honour your opponent. Since judo is by definition a spiritual and mental discipline, rather than merely a combat technique, the opponent is always held in esteem and his safety guarded. None the less, because of the constant grappling with an opponent and the large emphasis placed on competitive interaction, the risk of injury is high. This usually takes the form of strained joints, muscle pulls, particularly in back, arms and legs, as well as occasional breaks due to ill-timed falls.

In one way, judo is the most Westernized of the martial arts. It was established by Kano as an overtly competitive and sparing system of training. As such it has fitted very easily into the twentieth century paradigm of sports and competition. A precise system was established by Kano for scoring different throws, blows, and pins which has allowed it to be judged and winners elected. It was hence easily absorbed by Western athletes and particularly American soldiers after the war. In addition, Kano developed a ranking system which has since been simplified into different grades of belts, from white, then yellow, to brown and black, and then different stages or *dan* of black belt. Martial arts purists regret the co-option of judo into the competitive sporting world and the resultant loss in the philosophical underpinnings of non-aggression, defensiveness and physical and moral education.

As a physical discipline, judo demands a considerable degree of strength. It also requires flexibility and suppleness as you grapple in a wide variety of positions. While it lacks the lightning blows of karate, tae kwon do and Shaolin boxing, it does require quick reflexive responses as you seek both to maintain your balance and upset your opponent.

As well as flexibility, judo requires a good deal of strength training. Because it resembles Western wrestling in demands upon the body, it almost exclusively requires ATP and lactic acid energy systems to provide the necessary power. In addition, you must be constantly aware of the centre of balance and the use of your energy so that balance and contact with the ground is established. While all the martial arts systems emphasize balance and alignment, judo, in particular, requires these qualities in order to acquire the necessary skill. Because of the push and pull dynamic of the attempts to unbalance the opponent, a constant consciousness of one's central axis and weight are essential. Posture is emphasized precisely because one has to know how to maintain both a stable equilibrium and yet move quickly in towards one's central axis to make pivoting movements for throws and quick turns to resist an opponent's attempts to unbalance you.

Judo, along with aikido, is meant to be an effective system for smaller and less powerful people. Because the system is based upon gaining a lower centre of gravity, small individuals can often unbalance otherwise more powerful opponents. So judo, perhaps more than any other martial art, is practised by all age groups from children to grannies.

Judo, alone of the martial arts, is classified as a sport and hence included in Olympic and international competitions. Because of this there are fairly high standards of training and a systematic approach almost wherever you might choose to practise. Its family and sporting appeal gives it that extra bit of friendly and supportive atmosphere missing from the other major contact martial arts like karate, kung fu, tae kwon do. And since it does not involve striking techniques, it also appeals to women more than some of the other martial arts systems.

Like all martial arts, judo provides a powerful vehicle for fulfilling one's needs for achievement and perfection. In addition, many people find it a good balance between the softer martial arts (t'ai-chi and, to some extent, aikido) and the harder arts (karate, tai kwon do and kung fu). It is a middle path towards self-mastery.

Karate

Karate inspires visions of hand-chopping men shouting 'Ki-ae!' as they land fatal blows on their opponents. It is in fact the most popular martial art in Britain and is often pictured in books and magazines. It developed on the island of Okinawa, particularly during the seventeenth century when weapons of any kind were banned by the Japanese conquerors, and *kara-te* or 'empty hand' began to develop.

Karate is very physically demanding both from the point of view of the requirements of the body and the approach to training. Practice takes the form of the repetition of 'katas', or formalized attacking and defensive routines which are repeated again and again. There is a strong emphasis on the fundamentals in their repetition and you progress slowly through different katas as your ability improves. In attack the hand and foot, including the elbow and knee, are primarily used. There is more use of the upper body than in tae kwon do, and jumps are not as high.

As always there are a large number of different schools, reflecting the fact that for 300 years karate was an underground practice. You might hear of some of the older schools, the Shuri-te, Naha-te or Tomari-te schools from three different Okinawan cities in the nineteenth century. But more likely you will encounter one of three or four major schools. Of the two main Okinawan and hence more traditional schools, the Shorin-ryu or 'flexible pine school' uses light, fast movements and the stance is fairly high. There are several different styles in this school. The other is the Goju-ryu or 'hard and soft school'. Arm and leg movements are more circular and bent and there is a greater emphasis on breathing techniques.

The third commonly found school known as the Shotokan school was started by an Okinawan called Funakoshi Gichin. He was invited to Tokyo in 1922 to give a demonstration after the Emperor Hirohito saw an exhibition in Okinawa. He taught in Japan for some time and karate was taken up by the Japanese systematically over the next 20 years. Since the re-emergence of martial arts in Japan after the post-war ban, Shotokan karate has become more competitive and is used in sporting matches and sparring. This is a recent development which the purist karate masters and teachers regret. The form tends to be more angular and some people would suggest that there is less emphasis on the fundamentals of breath, posture and kata. Be that as it may, it is certainly a popular and major form of karate. Two other schools derived from the Japanese assimilation are the Wado-ryu and the Shito style.

Karate does not make reference to any of the animal forms which seem to enliven much of the Chinese martial traditions, particularly the Shaolin boxing and kung fu approaches. This undoubtedly reflects its lack of connection to the Taoist tradition and through it to the forces of nature and the Taoist conceptions of energy and flow. Indirectly, though Okinawan in origin, it has assumed closer connections with the Zen traditions of Japan and focuses, therefore, on strict codes and training regimes.

The Japanese and Okinawan forms do differ amongst themselves. Because of the Japanese penchant for competition and grading (witness the development of judo as a competitive sport), Japanese styles involve more sparring between partners and regular competitions. The Okinawan forms focus more on the artistic side, the discipline of oneself and self-growth. Depending upon your personal goals you may find yourself drawn towards either the more competitive or the more self-disciplined forms.

In training sessions students will spend a long time before doing the katas in a systematic warm-up. Because of the strenuous nature of the actual training session this is advisable. Systematic stretching of all the major muscles of the body and range of motion exercises to free and limber up the joints are carried out. Breathing exercises are also taught to be performed in conjunction with the katas. In most of the schools there is a definite emphasis on abdominal breathing rather than chest or upper body breathing. Focusing on the *tan-tien* or *hara* and through this centering are included in basic training.

Karate places great emphasis on strength training. In most karate dojos there is usually a variety of pieces of equipment for strengthening the muscles in the body, particularly those of the hands. This reflects the emphasis on the use of the upper body and the hands as the main attacking instruments. Special weights akin to dumb-bells are used to strengthen the fingers. They are grasped from one end with the fingers in a claw-like fashion and carried around the room. There are jars full of sand into which the hands are repeatedly plunged to strengthen and toughen the fingers. Some dojos will have padded wooden posts for practising against in a way that a boxer might practise with a punch bag. All of this training equipment is designed to toughen the physical body so that the karateka can deliver telling blows and can equally withstand those of his opponent.

Coordination is also of importance in karate, but because of the emphasis on power and strength you may find that neuro-muscular coordination is included in the practice of the katas but is restricted to the performance of the kata proper. Karate is known for its power as opposed to its grace or agility.

In addition to strength training there is direct emphasis given to posture and alignment. Specific exercises are prescribed to improve stance, positioning and balance. Emphasis is also placed on vertical alignment and hence the noticeably upright position and straight back which characterizes most karateka. Though this can seem wooden in newcomers, in the long term it results in a stable upright posture.

Like all martial arts, karate enhances your overall sense of well being. Because karate places so much emphasis on strength training it is going to result in more development of muscular power, but it does work with general joint flexibility as well. Karate dojos tend to be fairly rigorous and serious; while there is a fraternity between students, it does not have the same general ambience as some of the more social martial arts like judo or aikido. Emphasis is definitely on self-mastery and achievement of the katas.

Tae Kwon Do

Tae kwon do is the best known of the Korean martial arts. There are other variations like tae kwonpup, tae kwon, kwonpup, t'ang-su and subak but they all derive from the Korean tradition of empty handed fighting. Tae kwon do is a system which employs strikes and kicks almost to the exclusion of other techniques. There is no grappling as with judo or throwing as with aikido. Its name means literally the way of kicking with feet and destroying with hand.

Though there has been a definite influence by the hard Chinese tradition, Korea has always maintained its separate identity in martial arts throughout its history. No other martial art system relies so heavily upon the use of the feet. Many of the high jumps and kicks which typify this martial art are unique to it and it is thought by some experts that a number of the jumps Bruce Lee incorporated into his system of kung fu, were derived from tae kwon do techniques.

While the legs are probably not as fast as the arms and so delivery of a kick takes more time than a punch, the legs are longer and, as a result, kicks can be delivered to an oponent out of reach of one's arms. The potential strength of the kick is also greater than that of the punch. The danger stressed in tae kwon do training is that the kicks leave you unbalanced and in a vulnerable position. Thus some of the beautiful high-jumping kicks we have all admired in Bruce Lee films would never be used in normal combat because of the risk to counter attack they involve.

But tae kwon do is not just kicking. It is characterized by a wide range of strikes and blows using all and any parts of the body. There are a large number of hand movements many of which are similar to typical curving or circling hand techniques found in Chinese kung fu systems. There is an equal emphasis on defence and attack. Blocking, dodging and parrying techniques employing both hands and feet are taught. In addition, breathing techniques are strongly emphasized, coordinating the breathing with one's attacks and defensive manoevres. Energy gathering techniques are taught and a major one, *jiptjung* (power gathering), employs the breath.

There are set training forms which resemble the karate katas. But they tend to be less long or ritualized. There is an emphasis as well on training with sparring partners which employs body contact in a carefully supervised fashion. In sparring one also practises against armed opponents.

While tae kwon do employs very few of what may be considered the 'soft discipline' techniques, there is a strong moral code, very much like the *Budo* tradition in Japan. The thinking of the tae kwon do student is cultivated through the martial art; the way one thinks in the dojo is meant to set the pattern for how one approaches life. Discipline in the dojo and during the training regimes is strict. With the emphasis on breathing and some of the internal strengthening techniques, some affinity with the soft systems is implicit.

Tae kwon do places considerable emphasis on physical strength. The entire body is trained as much as possible so as to be able to perform the powerful, explosive jumps, kicks and punches. The wide range of movement demanded from the lower as well as the upper body results in considerable flexibility of all four limbs.

Because of the number of jumping and kicking movements, tae kwon do requires a fairly high degree of balance and stability. Good postural habits are learned because the individual becomes aware of his posture in a wide range of dynamic movements. Posture is maintained not as a rigid alignment of the body (as happens some times in karate) but as a sense of equilibrium throughout the complete range of positions, some of which are highly unstable. The result is an innate sense of balance and composure in whatever position one may find oneself.

As in most martial arts, the dojo is also a place of study. Tae kwon do takes itself seriously and the training attitude is one of discipline and hard work. Self-mastery as a personal goal is well and truly cultivated. It is one of the more physical martial arts and so if you are considering pursuing a martial discipline for self-expression or perhaps social reasons, you might consider judo or aikido. Tae kwon do can be physically gruelling, but it is a total body training and its acrobatic nature is a prime attraction for many.

Aikido

The Japanese word *aikido* is made up of three characters: *ai* meaning harmony or meeting; *ki* which is translated as energy, spirit, essence or breath; and *do* which means path or way. So *aikido* can be translated roughly as 'the way of divine harmony'. Like other Japanese martial arts it has its roots in the tradition of *Budo*, 'Way of the Warrior'. A relatively new art, it derives a considerable amount of its technical repertoire from a preceding system of specialized combat known as aiki-ju-jutsu, 'the flexible combat art of divine harmony'. This system of unarmed combat was characterized by the use of circular movements and a number of ensnaring techniques.

In 1917 a student with exceptional potential was given his teaching licence in aki-ju-jutsu. His name was Ueshiba Morihei. He had studied not only aiki-ju-jutsu but had devoted himself to mastering a number of other martial art forms, as well. In 1925, after many years of devoted training and study, he had a spiritual experience which transformed his perception of martial arts and *budo*:

> *Budo* is not felling the opponent by our force; nor is it a tool to lead the world into destruction with arms. True *Budo* is to accept the spirit of the universe, keep the peace of the world, correctly produce, protect and cultivate all beings in nature.

He took another dozen years reflecting upon and refining this perception and finally in 1938 began to teach aikido, 'the way of divine harmony'.

As a martial art, aikido is an art of self-defence. The goal of aikido is to control one's attacker not by conflicting with him, but rather by blending with him and redirecting the force of his attack. Almost all of the movements are circular, generally leading back to the aggressor. Thus it is not necessary to exert great strength to protect oneself from attack. To be able to redirect an opponent's attack, aikidoists must maintain a calm, peaceful state of mind. Aikido resonates with the soft martial arts tradition of China, so that whilst on the surface it bears little resemblance to t'ai-chi or pa-kua, it is essentially in harmony with the spirit of these and other forms of the inner school of martial arts.

The techniques of redirection are called *wazas*. They are

practised repetitively as are katas in karate schools. There are between fifty and one hundred different wazas and thousands of variations on them. They are all characterized by circular motions, which arise as a defensive response to an attack. Movement is centred on the hips. As an individual progresses in skills he will practise against an opponent with a wooden sword called a *bokken* and ultimately a four foot long staff which is called a *jo*.

Much emphasis is placed on understanding the nature of *ki*, (energy), and its flow, and ultimately experiencing this flow in and through you. Some schools of aikido place an even more particular stress on *ki* and teach what they call ki-aikido.

High levels of proficiency in aikido, and comprehension of the flow of *ki* as it moves through oneself and one's opponent culminates in what is known as the 'touchless throw', in which the aggressor is led to throw himself without being touched by the other. Ueshiba was famous for his touchless throws and being able to ward off five, six or more simultaneous attackers with apparent effortlessness. But Ueshiba contended that it is possible with aikido principles to control and redirect another's aggression before it ever reaches a state of conflict:

> When an enemy tries to fight me he has to break the harmony of the universe. Hence at the moment he has the mind to fight with me, he is already defeated.

Thoughts of competition, anger, aggression are all counter-productive to being in balance with the divine harmony and hence discouraged in aikido training. Ueshiba himself established aikido training along classical lines with no sparring or competitive elements. However a number of his students have established schools in which competitive approaches are taught and practised. The most well known of these schools was established by Tomiki, one of Ueshiba's students who had also studied judo with Kano. Tomiki-style aikido schools now flourish along with the more traditional, non-competitive forms.

Through the practice of aikido one learns to harmonize effort with the flow of energy by a constant focusing on one's centre of gravity (*hara*). Flexibility is also improved through practice of aikido forms and general body conditioning results from aikido practice. Endurance training is minimal as is the case with most martial arts, but a great deal of attention is placed on being relaxed and calm while practising so as to be able to remain in harmony with the flow of *ki*.

Aikido is one martial art which is based completely upon the principles of self-defence. In traditional Aikido training there are no attacking moves. In addition, because the emphasis is placed on effortless movement, on redirecting the energy of one's attacker, and on circular motions operating from the principle of defence, it is possible for individuals of all ages, whatever their physical makeup, to practise the art. Like t'ai-chi it can be taught almost as a movement awareness technique where the combative and aggressive elements of the martial arts tradition are minimalized. But, also like t'ai-chi, a deep tradition of discipline and physical, mental, emotional and spiritual training underlies aikido as a solid foundation and at its core it is a pure martial art system. The true masters and long-time students of aikido are as deft, powerful and self-controlled as any of the exponents of the harder and external forms of the martial arts.

Movement Awareness Techniques

Why, when the exercise systems, dance methods, sports and martial arts are themselves confusing enough, should we take the trouble to explore techniques with such exotic names as Eutony, Feldenkrais and Alexander?

The first and best reason lies in the ability of these movement awareness systems to promote well being, health, and in general to raise the overall level of awareness of the individual. Furthermore, movement awareness techniques can greatly enhance your performance in the more traditional exercise activities like sport and dance. It is common to find, for example, an ultra-distance runner in a yoga class, a golfer going to Alexander lessons, martial artists turning to Feldenkrais, swimmers doing a course in Eutony, or dancers in a Pilates studio. Thirdly, these movement systems are actually therapeutic: functional disorders, back problems, training injuries, osteoarthritic conditions, can all be greatly improved by the practice of one or more of these systems of movement. Finally, most have as their prime concern the cultivation of ease and pleasure. When practised sensibly students find a sense of communing with their body, of effortless movement, a sense of ease and of grace which brings a tremendous sense of satisfaction, calm and fulfilment.

Many of the contemporary movement awareness techniques, with the notable exception of yoga, trace their origins back to either the early dance pioneers or to the nationalistic developers of gymnastics and physical education in the eighteenth and nineteenth centuries. But the approach of the twentieth century saw the beginning of serious questioning in Europe of the militaristic form of fitness training developed by Gutsmuth,

Ling and Jahn. The strict conformity to prescribed routines, the military tradition and purpose, the intolerance of individual differences and capabilities, and an increasing awareness that the human body was a much more subtle and fascinating creation than had ever before been conceived, led to a number of physical educators, gymnastics teachers, physiotherapists, musicians, dancers and educators to question the whole premise upon which traditional physical training was based.

Jacques Dalcroze, a music teacher, conductor and student of Bruckner, developed what he called Eurythmic Education, based upon his teaching experience at the Geneva conservatory. He observed that his students did not really 'feel' the music in their bodies, but rather tried to recreate the beat through listening, tapping their feet or waving their arms. Dalcroze started to teach them to walk in time with the music, to move with it. What he discovered was that not only did their performance as musicians and conductors improve but through these movements they began to experience themselves as a whole entity. They connected with their identity as individuals. Dalcroze established a teaching centre in Germany to which many famous actors, musicians and performers came before it was interrupted by the Second World War. After the war, he returned to Geneva, where he opened the Institut Dalcroze which is still in operation.

Working more directly with the mainstream of dance, Rudolph von Laban developed his psychological and therapeutic interest in Germany during the 1930s. He was already an influential and leading figure in the arts and was choreographer of the Berlin Opera House and at Bayreuth. It was during this time that he began to study workers' movements, a study he continued when he later came to England, making a great contribution to movement psychology with special reference to industry. Laban also developed the first really viable dance notation, Labanotation, which is still widely used today. With Lisa Ullman, first in Manchester then in Surrey and finally London, Laban established the now world famous Laban Centre for Movement and Dance, where students can study every aspect of dance, movement theory and choreography.

Laban's principles of movement underlie the system of strength training developed by Joseph Pilates which uses a wide range of equipment, machines and power building exercises gaining in popularity today (see page 281).

The third stream of alternate approaches to movement arose through Elsa Gindler and her eventual collaboration with Heinrich Jacoby. Elsa Gindler was born in the 1880s and was trained as a physical education teacher. In 1910, when still in her early twenties, she contracted tuberculosis, and was advised by her doctors to retreat to the Swiss Alps. But being the daughter of working class parents, this was unfeasible, and so, like a number of other movement pioneers, she set about curing herself. She began by cultivating her sensitivity to her own inner functioning to the point where she was able to differentiate the breathing in her right lung from that in her left. She developed such acute sensitivity to her breathing that she was able to cease automatic interference with her organism's innate tendencies to regeneration by actually resting the infected lung and so facilitate its healing. She returned to her doctor a year later with, to his amazement, a complete remission of the disease. Inspired by her own self-transformation, she began to teach her *Arbeit am Menschen* (work on the human being) or *Nachenfaltung* (unfolding afterwards) as she later called her work.

In the early 1930s she began her collaboration with another pioneer in human learning and creativity, Heinrich Jacoby. Jacoby ran classes in movement, acting, improvisation and creativity in Zurich. He had a conviction that the way children spontaneously learn to talk is the prototype of all organic learning. Gindler and Jacoby collaborated for nearly thirty years, until her death in 1961. In their work the body's functioning took precedence over large, powerful or rapid movements, and it developed into a most subtle and gentle method of learning in which goal-orientated behaviour was restricted in favour of body awareness.

Concurrent to the work being done by Gindler and Jacoby, an Australian actor by the name of Matthias Alexander found that he began to lose his voice during his one-man recitals. Just as with Gindler, Alexander set about to find out what his affliction was and how to cure it. Through meticulous self-scrutiny, he learned to correct his problem and went on to teach a whole form of postural alignment and movement which organized itself around the correct initiation of movement from the head in a forward and upward motion (see pages 271–274). Alexander worked with scores of actors, musicians, celebrities and statesmen, and became one of the best known of the therapeutic movement pioneers.

Bess Mensendieck was born in the 1860s in America but gained her first insight into human movement when taking sculpture classes in Amsterdam. She began to notice how even individuals chosen as models for their aesthetic physical appearance still had poor coordination, flabby muscles and suffered from aches and pains. This memory stuck with her as she studied medicine in Zurich to become one of the first women doctors. Her desire to educate people in proper physical training technique led her to develop her Mensendieck System of Exercises. These resemble traditional exercises and some contemporary keep fit systems more than most awareness systems, but the emphasis is on cultivation of correct posture and range of movement. The exercises are usually gentle and are designed to introduce the participant to his body. Mensendieck uses the word 'shape' rather than train when talking of the effect of the exercises. The method is based on muscle function, and every exercise is carefully devised to provide the appropriate action that each muscle needs to keep in optimum health. Although the method never found wide acceptance in her native USA, it became very popular in Scandinavia where today a Mensendieck teacher has the same status as a physiotherapist, the one preventative, the other curative.

Whereas Western forms of movement learning and awareness techniques have only recently really begun to find their public, Eastern forms of training and meditational movement have been widely accepted for some time. No longer exotic, something for the eccentrics and post-hippies, yoga is probably the most familiar system of educating the body towards wellness, balance and awareness practised today throughout the West. It has also been the subject of scientific studies and research and is undoubtedly the basis of most forms of stretching now practised by sports people.

The work of Mabel Ellsworth Todd, stands out on two counts. Professor Todd taught movement education at Columbia University in New York. She taught posture and alignment to movement and PE teachers but placed considerable emphasis on the body as an organism in which opposing forces were constantly being kept in equilibrium. The potential for balance had to be inherent in the body in order for it to

function – walking, sitting, standing, crawling, even lying require a constant balancing of different forces.

As Professor Todd writes: 'The mechanisms for breathing,
locomotion, and mechanical balance are deeply tied in all the
bodily tissues, and structural adaptations for these functions are
closely interrelated.' Professor Todd pioneered substantial
work on the interrelationship of structure and function. Posture
and alignment were focused on in a way which makes them
comprehensible as a function of movement rather than of static
positions. Her work had a formative influence on many dancers,
particularly those who evolved Contact Improvization and
release work (see pages 233–236).

All of these early pioneers were breaking with the mould,
establishing other priorities in movement education besides
those of the gymnast, the physical educators and the military.
The emphasis began to shift from doing to being, from achieving goals to becoming aware of what you are doing to get there.
Power and strength began to take a back seat to awareness and
control. Endurance had also to allow for correct posture and
alignment. Conformity was replaced by spontaneity, creativity
and individual expression. Human beings were suddenly
allowed to be different from each other, to have idiosyncratic
movement patterns, to orchestrate a delicate counterbalance of
forces and to be rich with sensory experience and perception.

This refinement and cultivation of human sensory awareness
through movement has grown and expanded throughout the
latter half of the twentieth century as students of the early
pioneers and new explorers have become better known. Moshe
Feldenkrais, a judo black belt and research physicist, developed
a system which allows for a complete re-education of the human
nervous system and the interruption of counterproductive
movement patterns (see pages 274–278). Charlotte Selver and
Charles Brooks have refined the work of Elsa Gindler in their
teaching of Sensory Awareness, to the point where Alan Watts,
philosopher and the most famous advocate in the West of Zen
meditation, was moved to exclaim after experiencing their
work: 'But this is living Zen!' In Sensory Awareness classes
movement itself is restricted to the point where awareness of the
body is the sole objective. Standing, sitting, lying, walking,
touching, contact with others, contact with the environment
become the focus for awareness. The senses take the fore-

ground.

Gerda Alexander, long-time student of Jacques Dalcroze, developed her system called Eutony (see page 278) in which the focus of awareness shifts to the tonus of the musculature.

Lulu Sweigard, student and colleague of Mabel Todd, refined nine major lines of movement where repeated unconscious contractions result in structural imbalance and postural defects. And she developed a system which is more effective at interrupting the chronic contractions along those lines of movement than therapeutic manipulation. Dancers all over America use her ideokinetic imaging techniques to help them put into action the true intention of their movements (see Posture pages 128–138).

One difficult decision in writing about awareness techniques was to exclude t'ai-chi from this section and place it instead with the martial arts. Although it derives very firmly from the martial arts tradition, as it is currently practised today it deserves to be considered as a prime movement awareness technique. Its benefits for postural correction are substantial. And importantly it cultivates correct movement and range of movement in the joints in an upright position so that therapeutic benefits are available in daily life. It is seldom practised in its martial form except by its most advanced students.

The inclusion of movement awareness systems in a book on exercise reflects that this formerly esoteric pursuit of awareness through movement is no longer a sideline to the main stream of movement and exercise. In the same way that complementary healing methods are now becoming widely accepted and their practitioners highly trained, in the same way as good diet and nutrition are now becoming central concerns for anyone actively involved in improving their physical health and well being, so too, new systems of therapeutic movement and conscious education of the control system of the body are coming to the foreground as essential elements of the changing consciousness people are experiencing. Bodies are being raised from their status as a 'thing' or 'object'. People are beginning to realise that a positive, loving and caring relationship with their physical being does as much as anything towards cultivating health, enjoyment, well being and longevity. Regular practice of a movement awareness technique results in an enhanced self-image, an increase in the ease and efficiency of movement and general emotional stability and happiness. Finally, movement awareness techniques seem to help us discover more of who we are and how we regulate our physical being in order to express our inner potential in a balanced and harmonious fashion.

Yoga

Hatha Yoga is the most ancient form of body conditioning now practised and its postures are the single greatest influence on all the Western systems designed for flexibility and suppleness.

Yoga has been practised in the West since the nineteenth century and in its country of origin, India, for over 3000 years. Its popularity has grown with steady regularity, ignoring trends, fads and hype, and there are now thousands of yoga teachers and many more practitioners in every country in the West. In fact, it is probably fair to say that it is easier to find a good yoga teacher in many small towns than a good teacher of a Western keep fit method.

There are three key aspects which make for yoga's high quality and consistent appeal as a method of exercising the body: the meticulousness of the postures which stretch and tone every part of the body, the emphasis on non-competitiveness and relaxation, and lastly the philosophy and total approach to life that is offered. These three aspects, taken together, also make yoga the original movement awareness technique. It is impossible to practise yoga well without concentration and awareness, and the emphasis on slow, quiet movement, on really feeling that turn in the thigh or reach of the shoulder joint, gradually builds up a heightened attention and a sense of one's body, inside and out, which is deeply satisfying.

The physical practice of yoga, which is what is meant by the term Hatha Yoga, consists of two parts: the asanas (postures) and pranayama (breathing exercises). Some schools emphasize one more than the other, but a combination of both is essential. The asanas are not exercises as such but precisely defined postures which the student moves into and then holds for as long as he can. The better you get, the longer you hold them. There are hundreds of asanas. Some focus on a specific area of the body – a limb, joint, muscle group. Others are designed to stimulate different internal organs or body systems. There are groups of asanas which aid digestion, prevent constipation, improve circulation, strengthen the stomach or pelvic floor, and so on. In the average class only a proportion of these are practised, usually in a balanced combination of standing postures, sitting poses and twists and lying poses, ending with the shoulder stand and finally relaxation.

There are fewer breathing exercises (pranayama), about 15–20, and a selection of these are done either at the beginning of the class, at the end, during, or incorporated into the asanas, according to the practices of the different schools. Again these aim to improve breathing, lung capacity, concentration and awareness, as well as providing the benefits to the rest of the body of deep, regular respiration. This emphasis on the breath is crucial, and correct breathing during movement (out on the effort, in on the return) is often sorely lacking in modern keep fit systems. Breathing properly during exercise also increases one's physical power and ability to perform a movement with ease and balance. *Prana* means life force and is the correlate of the Chinese *chi*; it is the source of energy and also its manifestation in the body. When we focus on the breath we turn our attention inwards and become more aware of our centre, that point, just above the solar plexus, which should be the source of action.

There is a no nonsense, no glitter, no frills style to yoga. While there can be laughter and shared fun in a yoga class there is a level of absorption that is usually found only in movement awareness or professional dance classes, rarely in other forms of exercise or keep fit. The training that yoga teachers undergo is still one of the most rigorous: generally about three years of practical, theoretical and teaching practice. Such a course does not attract the fly-by-nighters so you can expect your yoga teacher to know what she or he is talking about and to convey that knowledge well. The theoretical part of the training deals with a knowledge of anatomy and the working of the body, and also requires study of the philosophical base of yoga.

Yoga means to join – our word to yoke comes from it. Hatha Yoga, the yoga of physical development, is one stage in the development of the whole person towards a higher plane. According to the ancient classical texts, the Upanishads, the Vedas, the Yoga Sutras, and the Hatha Yoga Pradipika, from which our knowledge of yoga comes (and which a yoga teacher must study), the essence of yoga is to attain, via the body, a state of inner peace and thus self-realization.

There are four main paths of yoga: that of action, of devotion, of knowledge and wisdom, and of physical and mental control. Each path is said to appeal to individuals of a different nature: all lead to the same goal of inner peace and enlightenment. Hatha Yoga is a subdivision of the last path, Raja Yoga, that of physical and mental control. Raja Yoga itself is divided into eight steps designed to refine and develop the individual.

The average practitioner of yoga is generally hardly aware of the rich philosophical and spiritual culture which underlies the physical movement – or even wants to be. Some of the foremost yogis (who are not extraordinary creatures capable of eating glass or walking on coals, but simply revered masters of yoga) have come over the years to the West, and adapted the practice and Indian philosophy in accordance with Western expectations to provide an accessible movement and health system. Yogis such as B.K.S. Iyengar, who put great emphasis on the correct performance of the asanas, and the physical force required, and Vishnu Devananda, who emphasized the role of relaxation, diet and positive attitude, with meditation along with the postures, for an all-round approach, have done a great deal to popularize yoga in the West. By playing down the spiritual aspects they have attracted thousands of ordinary people keen to take care of their bodies and develop flexible limbs and supple minds, but perhaps suspicious of a culture and religion so foreign to their own. Today, however, more people are showing an interest in this side of yoga, and more are acknowledging the value of the yogic approach in conjunction with the physical.

Yoga practice has been characterized as the relationship between physical body and conscious spirit with the mind as catalyst. For the mind to create that link, it must be focused, and so discipline and concentration are marked characteristics of a yoga class. While competitiveness is never encouraged, the emphasis on performing the asanas correctly can inevitably lead to some competitiveness. It is left to the individual to be aware of this danger, to stop when a pose becomes too hard to maintain and to be aware of what is happening with his or her own body rather than look at others. The plus side of the effort put into the asanas, some of which are very difficult and can take years to master, is the atmosphere of group support. In this context, the role of relaxation in yoga is a key one, both during the exercises when you allow your body to 'relax into' the pose, and at the end of the class, when you lie for between 5–15 minutes in what is known as the corpse pose.

Yoga is a relatively static exercise form. Those who need and enjoy more free-flowing movement may find this aspect frustrating. Yoga is excellent for flexibility and improved breathing rather than cardiovascular training.

There are several different schools of yoga with teachers spread all over Britain. Each has a slightly different emphasis or approach while the basic asanas and pranayama exercises will be the same. Different approaches will appeal to different people and it is a matter of trial and error to find one that suits you.

The Alexander Technique

The Alexander Technique, named after its creator, an Australian called F. Matthias Alexander, is an approach to therapeutic movement which works on internal cues and self-regulation. This makes it hard to describe to those who have not done it. As in most of the awareness methods it places a tremendous emphasis on listening to the body and picking up subtle clues from the proprioceptive nerves and the kinaesthetic sense. Of all the movement systems described in this book, it is the one which has the least 'movement' in it. The sessions are conducted on a one-to-one basis and the individual is moved or guided through certain positions rather than making the movements on his own. As one of the earliest of the modern movement re-education techniques to develop in the West, it lays justifiable claim to being one of the grandfathers of the movement awareness world. At the same time it suffers somewhat from the limiting bias of its early development; some consider the technique to be too rigid and prescribed, while others swear by it.

Like most movement awareness techniques this one grew out of personal problems. A bright child, brought up in a remote Tasmanian outpost, Alexander was a passionate admirer of Shakespeare and the theatre. By the age of 19 he was reciting in the theatres of Melbourne. It was here that his troubles started: he began to lose his voice during performances. His condition grew progressively worse until he had to walk out in the middle of performances, having completely lost his voice. Doctors could offer no help.

Like most people who have managed to overcome severe difficulties and break damaging patterns by discovering new approaches, Alexander did not take his impediment sitting down. He spent years studying what it was that he did to himself to cause the loss of voice and what he needed to do to recover it. He discovered that he had been pulling his head backwards and downwards immediately before he began to speak. The process whereby he made this discovery and learnt how to interrupt his bad habit formed the basis of a system of movement education to which he dedicated the rest of his life.

The basic prime cause of the misuse of the body as seen from the Alexander viewpoint is this pulling down and backwards of the head, which during the course of hundreds of movements each day compresses the spine and pulls it slowly out of alignment. The effect is impaired movement, distorted proprioceptive information from the neck, inner ears and ultimately the rest of the body. The end result is compression of the chest, ribs and spine, causing inefficient functioning of the internal organs, circulation and a general lessening of the overall health of the body. Through lessons in the technique, you discover that this is only one of a series of bad habits which we are liable to develop in the use of ourselves during our lives. The Alexander Technique aims to untangle these bad habits so that movement becomes effortless and smooth. Alexander preferred not to consider his work as therapeutic; he called his patients 'students' and he preferred lessons to be considered as reconditioning processes not exercises.

There are several key concepts in the Alexander Technique. One of them is the concept of 'use'. 'Right' or 'good' use means moving the body with coordination and balance, so that only the effort necessary to produce the movement is expended. One never forces oneself into the 'correct' position because by definition you will then use extra muscle power to pull against unconsciously contracted muscles and therefore use more effort to keep yourself in alignment.

Alexander focused on the habitual movement patterns which we unconsciously slip into over the years when performing relatively simple, repetitive actions (such as walking, getting up from a chair, reading, writing or playing an instrument). His aim was to interrupt these habits and focus our attention on the movement process, not its end. This forms the basis of another key concept: 'the means whereby', which Alexander defines as 'the reasoned means to the gaining of the end'. In other words, in order to interrupt an old habitual pattern of movement you have to take your attention away from the ends and focus it on the means. The moment your concern is solely the *goal* of a particular movement you fall back into the old movement habits to achieve it. You take short cuts or use the most familiar pathway in the nervous system to accomplish the movement. Even if, as is often the case, this pattern is inefficient, or worse, counterproductive in terms of body usage, you will still follow it because it is familiar. After making you conscious of the bad habits the Alexander Technique replaces them with new movement patterns to enhance body functioning.

The technique may improve the functioning of your respiratory muscles through changing the muscle tone of the ribs and diaphragm, but there is no direct conditioning effect on either lungs or heart. Likewise it offers little in the way of strength training. Emphasis on these things is seen as 'end-gaining' so no attempt is made to build up muscle during lessons. There is no focus on flexibility since for Alexander 'right use' did not involve any particular emphasis on increasing the range of movement in the joints except in so far as this enhanced his postural teaching. It is in working with alignment and posture that the Alexander Technique is at its best, and it is found highly beneficial in those sports where alignment is crucial, such as in golf and riding. This technique moves right away from the dictates of military posture – chin in, chest forward, shoulders back – which have been the undoing of generations of 'well brought up' people. This was one of Alexander's most important innovations. Posture is a concept which is subsumed under 'right use'. It works with subtle proprioceptive cues and an enhanced kinaesthetic awareness of the use of the body. The forward and upward movement of the head works directly on a number of basic reflexes for organizing movement and keeping yourself in a vertical position. The Alexander Technique is particularly good at getting you to participate consciously in this process and yet not confusing you with too many 'shoulds' and 'oughts'.

Finally, the Alexander Technique is particularly valuable for neuromuscular education. While it may not necessarily improve the performance of a skill, nor help with anticipation (so essential in many sports), it does educate the participant to have a more direct relationship with the central nervous system. You will remember that analysis and thought about a movement comes from the motor cortex, the part of the brain involved in differentiating movement patterns, sorting through experience and experimenting with different variations or parts of the body. When a pattern is learned it is shifted to the premotor area of the brain: we don't think about moving, it just happens. What the Alexander Technique does is help to shift our awareness of our movements up to the motor cortex area so that we can begin to interrupt the unconscious habits of movement which are our everyday norm. So the student is helped to participate in creating change in bad habits and inefficient ways of moving, particularly as this relates to posture and alignment. Musicians and actors have been especially drawn to the technique, in part because of Alexander's own heritage. George Bernard Shaw, for example, was a great devotee. The strain of maintaining set positions when playing an instrument, causing chronic tension and postural imbalances, has led countless musicians to the technique as well.

Through the process of Alexander lessons, one begins to experience the good use of oneself, and bad usage and inappropriate habits begin to be slowly edged out until a more balanced and conscious use of the body becomes the norm.

The Feldenkrais Method

Like other awareness techniques, the Feldenkrais Method is based upon the research and work of one individual who confronted traditional methods of training the body and found them lacking. Moshe Feldenkrais was born in 1903 in a small village in western Russia. In his teens he emigrated to what was then Palestine, where he earned his livelihood through manual labour and through teaching self-defence to the Jewish population. In his twenties he was admitted to the Sorbonne where he eventually received his Doctorate of Science in physics and subsequently worked with Frédéric Joliot Curie in atomic physics. It was during his stay in France that he met Mr Kano, the founder of judo, who was so impressed with one of the books which Feldenkrais had written on self-defence that he invited him to the Japanese Embassy to demonstrate his technique. Feldenkrais went on to become one of the first Western black belts in judo and helped found the Judo Club de France. He wrote dozens of books on the subject.

In 1940 he was forced to flee the Nazi occupation and, carrying secret documents, made his way through the French Underground to Britain where he worked for the Ministry of Defence on submarine detection techniques. During this time he became involved with the Scottish Judo Association. But it was due to the flaring up of an old knee injury that he first began to explore the principles and ideas that form the basis of the work that takes his name. Doctors were pessimistic about the prognosis for his knee, relegating him to the future use of a cane. He rejected this prospect and immersed himself in the sciences of the body: anatomy, neurophysiology, kinesiology, biochemistry and anthropology. In 1947 he published the results of these studies in his book, *Body and Mature Behaviour*. He also amazed doctors and friends by restoring the function of his defective knee.

The Feldenkrais Method is not about fitness or physical training. It is about learning. The key to any kind of movement education lies in the ability to recognize what you are doing, how you are able to do it and how you can repeat the movement effortlessly and by choice. Unlike animals, whose behaviour is fundamentally predetermined by their nervous system (a new-born calf will stand within an hour of birth), almost all of our activity is learned. The way we sit, roll over, stand, eat, play a musical instrument, repair a watch or polevault 18 feet, all are learned.

'As a result man has both the extraordinary opportunity given to no other animal, to build up a body of learned response, *and* his special vulnerability of going wrong. Since other animals have their response to most stimulae wired into their nervous system in the form of instinctive patterns of activity, they go wrong less frequently. Even more irritating, we have little opportunity to become aware of where we went wrong since we are the learner and the judge at the same time. Our judgement depends on and is limited to our learned experience.'

In order to break this vicious circle, Feldenkrais developed over the years a large number (over 1000) of unique lessons which he called Awareness Through Movement. The lessons are conducted in a non-stressful environment at a slow pace. Many of the lessons take place in a lying, sitting or kneeling position. This facilitates the breakdown of unconscious muscular patterns starting with the habitual response of the anti-gravity muscles (see Posture, page 128). By making new or unusual movements in new and unusual positions, the nervous system must generate alternative solutions, which combine familiar movements with unusual or unfamiliar sensations. As a result awareness of how the body functions is enhanced and the individual begins to choose consciously how he or she moves.

Since the Feldenkrais Method is based on learning (learning to learn, in fact), the group classes in Awareness Through Movement are not based on goal-oriented behaviour – if anything, participants are asked to forego goals until they have a clear awareness of what they are doing. Habitual, unconscious patterns of movement are inhibited. Re-learning movement and acting through unconscious choice are encouraged.

Another key concept in the Feldenkrais Method is differentiation – the ability to break complex movement patterns down into components and then restructure them into new permutations and combinations as a part of the learning process. As such, Feldenkrais lessons keep you constantly working with your motor cortex, shifting learned patterns up into that part of the brain which allows you to interrupt older, learned habits. With Feldenkrais, however, there is no such thing as a 'right movement'. Rather each situation calls forth the appropriate movement from the body. It is only unconscious learned habits which we repeat again and again which restrict our movement potential.

Another way of looking at our use of ourselves is to consider how we began as an infant with a number of disparate bits and pieces: arms, legs, head, etc. Through use and experience we make connections between these body parts so that we learn how to lift a spoon to our mouth, scratch the back of our head, swim, run or swing a tennis racquet. Over our years of experience we explore a wide range of possible ways of performing these movements and accumulate the most commonly used movement combinations which meet our needs – that is, until you encounter a new or unusual request upon your body. Then, like a commuter who has only ever taken one route to work and one day finds it blocked, you suddenly find yourself unable to perform or accomplish your objective. You are unable to do what you want to do. Habitual movement patterns may work 70 or even 99 per cent of the time, but if you don't have alternative choices available in your nervous system then you are limited in your response to the world.

In Awareness Through Movement classes, patterns are differentiated and then re-assembled but there is always room left for exploration and experimentation. Through discovering new solutions to old goals, the Feldenkrais Method seeks to expand the potential range of movement so that one's body and control system can evoke the appropriate movement for each new situation rather than be limited to well-tried groups of habitual response. Feldenkrais puts it this way:

> Addressing the body to perfect all the possible forms and configurations of its members not only changes the strength and flexibility of the skeletal muscles but makes a profound change in the self image and the quality of direction of the self.

Implicit in this statement is the belief that after several million years of functional evolution, the body has the innate inner knowledge which will generate the appropriate movement for each situation if only we can begin to interrupt unconscious learned habits from past experience and choose consciously how we move.

The Feldenkrais Method does not offer much in the way of strength training and even less in terms of endurance. But it is one of the very best systems for increasing neuromuscular coordination. It also works substantially on the posture of the body. Of all the movement systems it is the easiest one in which to achieve relaxation whilst taking part in the classes. It also increases range of movement in the joints and so, while it does not increase flexibility to the same extent as yoga, it does improve the ability to use the wider range of movement of the joints which should be the major goal of flexibility training.

Like other awareness techniques, you can enter into a Feldenkrais class with no experience. Coordination skills are developed through the lessons themselves. The tempo and pace is very gentle and slow.

Feldenkrais lessons seem to complement a wide range of activities, and it is not uncommon to see a ballet dancer, a sportsman, a yoga teacher, an actor, a musician or a body conditioning teacher all in the same class. Because there is no competition in the classes it is possible to enter into a class and feel that you are a part of a group and you have similar goals to your fellow participants. Socializing is encouraged. There is also a sense of increased self-control and mastery as you begin to untie your movement knots and discover how to interrupt bad habits and unconscious patterns. Classes will also include participants who may have arthritic problems or who are recovering from physical injuries. Because of the nature of the lessons and the atmosphere of the classes, injuries are almost unknown and general well being and physical functioning is cultivated.

Eutony

Eutony is the name for a system of movement education developed by Gerda Alexander (no relation to Matthias of the Alexander Technique), who was born in Wuppertal, Germany, in 1908. Her parents were admirers of the teachings of Jacques Dalcroze and his Eurythmic Education and, as a child, Gerda Alexander was brought up under the principles of the Dalcroze system, learning how to feel music in the whole body – the rhythm, beat and pulse. Later she went on to teach eurythmics in Sweden and Denmark. It was in the 1930s that she started to develop her own form of movement education to which she gave the name Eutony. As she travelled to different schools of movement education she noticed something curious: the students of the different movement teachers (Wigman, Laban, Mensendieck, Gindler, Dalcroze) all developed movement characteristics typical of their group and their teacher. Though each system seemed valuable, their different styles suggested to

Alexander that there must be some simpler form of movement education that could precede them, linking their similarities.

The word Eutony is derived from the Greek *eu*, meaning good or harmonious, and *tonus* meaning tension. Together they describe a system of movement in which there is well balanced tension.

The ability to regulate tonus is the key to movement in Eutony. Each situation in life calls for a new and appropriate response: different levels of tonus for climbing stairs, playing tennis, walking on the beach, or dancing at the disco. It is the internal tonus which regulates our response to the outside world.

Alexander says that through a variety of situations – early childhood learning, school situations, repeated fearful experiences, etc – tonus can become fixed at a specific level in a part or all of the body. We can no longer regulate it in accordance with the requirements of each situation. Eutony helps the individual *learn* to regulate muscle tonus and so control of appropriate response through a number of different processes.

The beginner starts by developing his faculties and perception of his skin, weight, shape and boundaries of the body. There is ample time spent in classes feeling how the body makes contact with the surfaces of the floor, a wall or other objects. This is done both at rest and in movement. The skin is of vital importance in Eutony, and realizing and experiencing the boundary between yourself and your environment begins to give you a sense of your own self-image: what shape you actually are, how you are contained, how you differentiate yourself from other people and objects and in so doing discovering your three dimensional self-image. Dancers, for example, have a very two dimensional self-image because they work so much with mirrors. Most of us have large parts of our body for which we have a very limited self-image: our back, our buttocks, the sides of our rib cage, parts of our legs, and so forth. Time is spent in Eutony classes regaining a full, three dimensional self-image.

The second step in working with Eutony movements helps the individual to fill in the space between the side to side dimensions of the body. We have an inside as well as a surface. Through Eutony the sense of space inside us and how it is filled with muscles, organs and the skeletal structure (which is the basis of all movement) can be cultivated so that the student begins to judge for himself which muscles are chronically shortened or contracted, and which muscles are slack or underused. In Eutony classes a variety of 'control positions' are taught which allow the student to gauge the relative tonus of the different muscle groups and begin to feel the correct balance of tonus throughout the body.

Eutony works substantially with posture and alignment as well. Posture is aligned through working with the postural reflexes from the feet up to the head. Posture is examined in terms of how the individual transports the force of his own weight on his feet throughout the body, up through the pelvis and through the spine to the atlas vertebra at the base of the skull. Breathing is used only very gently, and never to force or speed up a process. There is no right way to breathe – a specific time to breathe in or out with movements – rather, breathing should be spontaneous and uninterrupted.

Gerda Alexander is very much opposed to aggressive systems of body work and to some extent physical fitness training. She speaks of a process of 'maturation' during which the individual increases self-awareness, sensitivity and self-mastery so that he becomes more present to himself and has a conscious relationship with his environment. The maturation of this experience results in a sense of self-expression and creativity as well as freedom of movement and a deep sense of well being. This allows the individual to choose his own mode of movement and expression without there being a right or a wrong way. Alexander likes to think that her students are all unique in their own expressions of who they are and have not just learned one form of movement training or the 'correct' way to move.

Eutony classes develop a high degree of sensitivity and hence an increase in neuromuscular awareness. While it does not work to the same degree as the Feldenkrais Method on neuromuscular control, sensory awareness is still central to the learning techniques employed. The movements in the classes are wide and varied: slow movements, rolling and floor work, stretching and some gentle strengthening, as well as standing and postural work are all included.

Relaxation is cultivated in the best possible way through the ability to regulate the level of tonus in the muscles. This is directly related to the control of the arousal levels of the body and the involuntary nervous system. Eutony is one of the best systems of training yourself to relax while moving: to utilize the minimal arousal and muscle tonus required to accomplish a task. It is excellent for stress reduction during work, exercise or daily life.

Like most awareness systems, it does very little for either strength or endurance training. It is excellent for posture and alignment and integrates the postural training into more movement and real-life situations than yoga, for example. Like the Feldenkrais Method, it incorporates its re-education of the nervous system into movement and coordination, making the learning applicable to life situations.

Classes are usually an hour long and it is possible to participate at any level of experience. Eutony is paricularly valuable to anyone whose job makes special demands upon their body: actors, musicians, dancers, sculptors and individuals with physical handicaps as well.

Pilates Technique

The Pilates Technique is fast being recognized in the UK as an economical and efficient method of body control and conditioning. It was developed by the late Joseph Pilates in America, where he had emigrated from his native Germany during the rise of Fascism.

Through meeting Rudolf von Laban in America, Pilates, already devoted to exercise, health and fitness, became even more concerned with the necessity for anatomical precision in exercise. As a result, the technique he developed has become one of the safest and most precise of the popular conditioning exercise forms around.

The basic format is the repetition of an individually devised routine of small, controlled, stretching and lifting exercises with the use of a number of simple machines and benches incorporating springs, harnesses, weights and moving parts. However, the emphasis is not on what you do but how you do it, and Pilates set forth eight basic principles which are constantly stressed in the teaching. These are: concentration, breathing, posture, centring, control, flowing movements, relaxation and stamina.

Students are individually taught and supervised at all times so studios and numbers are small, staff/client ratio high and safety record impeccable. The technique has become one of the most highly favoured for injury rehabilitation, particularly among dancers, as every body part can be isolated and exercised without stress on any other; all movements are smooth and rhythmic, and weights, balance and position are all adjustable to the needs of the individual.

Underlying the technique is the structure of Pilates' aims and philosophy, which are similar to the Eastern forms of movement and those of other re-education methods. Through regular training and attention to the eight basics the aim is to create a fusion of mind and body and a relaxed, balanced way of moving with economy, grace and strength. As a student you learn a great deal about how your body works, its strengths and weaknesses, how to correct its imbalances and use it to its full advantage.

Unlike some of the martial arts and movement awareness techniques, Pilates does not lay great emphasis on cultivating inner awareness and 'soft' energy. In line with dance technique there is a strong emphasis on developing the abdominal muscles as the central force from which exercises are performed and to breathe into the middle and upper lungs (keeping belly firm) rather than deep into the abdomen. Pilates recognized that strong abdominal muscles are essential for avoiding lumbar damage and injury to the back, but it is possible that in emphasizing upper chest breathing full development of the diaphragm is not allowed and a certain rigidity may be the result.

However, this method is proving to be an excellent introduction to body awareness in the context of the popular dance and exercise studios and has been drawing customers from the aerobics and mass exercise classes. The atmosphere in a Pilates studio is one of concentration and calm. Music, if any, is likely to be classical.

Sessions are booked and students follow their own routine in their own time at their own pace with a number of highly trained staff moving amongst the equipment adjusting the position of a thigh here, a weight there, judging a person's fatigue level or instructing a move to a different bench, giving reminders to breathe properly, dealing with problems, questions and details. Repetitions are kept to a maximum of sixteen to avoid boredom, and routines are devised to ensure a thoroughly balanced workout while suiting the needs of the individual. A session lasts for an hour and a half. While it may be strenuous, the end result is revitalizing since while the individual body part works the rest of the body is relaxed, and the concentration the student must bring to each movement, even to such a simple exercise as pulling the foot in a harness through a sprung slide at the right pace for the right number of times with the right turnout, ensures alertness and a sense of satisfaction. The physical results are invariably improved posture, line and muscle tone, greater flexibility and better placement, as well as greater awareness of breathing and balance.

Recommended Reading

Alexander, F. Matthias, *The Use of the Self* (Re-Educational Publ. Ltd, Weybridge, Surrey, 1955)

Anderson, Bob, *Stretching* (Shelter Publications, California, 1980)

Arnold, Peter J., *Meaning in Movement, Sport & Physical Education* (Heinemann, London, 1979)

Arnot, Dr Robert & Gaines, Charles, *Sports Selection* (The Viking Press, New York, 1984)

Astrand, P. O. & Rodahl, K., *Textbook of Work Physiology* (McGraw Hill, New York)

Baker, William J., *Sports in the Western World* (Rowman & Littlefield, Totowa, New Jersey, 1982)

Benson, Herbert, M. D., *The Relaxation Response* (Avon, New York, 1976)

Brooks, Charles V. W., *Sensory Awareness* (Ross-Erikson Publ., Santa Barbara, 1974)

Brown, Barbara B., *Stress and the Art of Biofeedback* (Bantam, New York, 1978)

Cannon, Geoffrey & Einzig, Hetty, *Dieting Makes You Fat* (Century, London, 1983)

Cooper, Kenneth, MD, *The Aerobics Way* (Corgi, London, 1978)

Diagram Group, The, *The Brain: A User's Manual* (Berkley Books, New York, 1984)

Dominguez, Richard H., M. D. & Gajda, Robert, *Total Body Training* (Warner Books, New York, 1983)

Draeger, Donn F. & Smith, Robert W., *Comprehensive Asian Fighting* (Kodansha International Ltd, Tokyo, 1983)

Dyer, K. F., *Catching Up the Men* (Junction Books, London, 1982)

Feldenkrais, Moshe, *Awareness through Movement* (Harper and Row International, New York, 1977); *Body & Mature Behaviour* (Universities Press Inc., New York, 1970)

Ferrucci, Piero, *What We May Be* (Turnstone Press, Northamptonshire, 1982)

Fonda, Jane, *Jane Fonda's Workout Book* (Simon & Schuster, New York, 1981)

Gaines, Charles & Butter, George, *Pumping Iron* (Sphere Books Ltd, London, 1977)

Gallwey, W. Timothy, *Inner Tennis* (Random House, New York, 1976)

Greene Morgan, Phyllis, *Dancercise* (Methuen, London, 1983)

Harrison, E. J., *Manual of Karate* (Sterling Publ., London, 1975)
Hutton, Deborah, (Ed.), *The Vogue Exercise Book* (Octopus Books, London, 1984)
Iyengar, B. K. S., *Light on Yoga* (Unwin Paperbacks, London, 1974)
Jacobson, Edmund, M. D., *You Must Relax* (McGraw-Hill Book Co., New York, 1978)
Kapit, Wynn & Elson, Lawrence, M., *The Anatomy Coloring Book* (Harper & Row, New York, 1977)
Klein, Bob, *Movements of Magic* [Tai Chi] (Newcastle Publ. Co. Inc., Hollywood, 1984)
Leggett, Trevor P. & Watanabe, K., *Championship Judo* (Foulsham, Slough, 1964)
Leonard, George, *The Ultimate Athlete* (Avon, New York, 1977)
Livet, Anne, (Ed.), *Contemporary Dance* (Abbeville Press, New York, 1978)
Lockhart, R. D., *Living Anatomy* (Faber & Faber, London, 1979)
McArdle, William D., Katch, Frank I. & Victor L., *Exercise Physiology* (Lea & Febiger, Philadelphia, 1981)
McConnell, Joan, *Ballet as Body Language* (Harper & Row, New York, 1977)
Morris, Alfred, F., *Sports Medicine* (W. C. Brown Publishers, Dubuque, Iowa, 1984)
Murphy, Michael & White, Rea, *The Psychic Side of Sports* (Addison-Wesley, California, 1978)
Murray, Jan, *Dance Now* (Penguin, London, 1979)
Newsholme, Eric & Leech, Tony, *The Runner* (Fitness Books, New Jersey)
Payne, Peter, *Martial Arts* (Thames & Hudson, London, 1981)
Reid, Howard & Croucher, Michael, *The Way of the Warrior* (Century, London, 1983)
Rosenweig, Sandra, *Sports Fitness for Women* (Harper & Row, New York, 1982)
Rowett, H. G. O., *Basic Anatomy and Physiology* (John Murray, London, 1983)
Sivananda Yoga Centre, *The Book of Yoga* (Ebury Press, London, 1983)
Solomon, Dr Henry, *The Exercise Myth* (Angus & Robertson, Sydney, 1984)
Sorenson, Jacki, *Aerobic Dancing* (Rawson, Wade Publ. Inc., New York, 1977)
Spino, Mike, *Beyond Jogging* (Celestial Arts, California, 1976)
Sweigard, Lulu E. PhD, *Human Movement Potential* (Harper & Row, New York, 1974)
Syer, John, *Team Spirit* (Heinemann 1986)
Syer, John & Connolly, Christopher, *Sporting Body Sporting Mind* (Cambridge University Press, Cambridge, 1984)
Todd, Mabel Elsworth, *The Thinking Body* (Dance Horizons Inc., New York, 1978)
Tohei, Koichi, *Aikido in Daily Life* (Japan Publications, Tokyo, 1973)
Turnbull, Alison, *Running Together* (Allen & Unwin, London, 1985)
Wehman, Morei Uyeshiba, *Aikido* (Hackensack, New Jersey, 1968)
Williams, Norma & Einzig, Hetty, *The New Guide to Women's Health* (Macdonald, London, 1985)

Useful Addresses

Aikido
British Aikido Board
6 Halking Croft, Langley, Slough, Berks
Tel. 75 73985

British Aikido Association
Atomace, Bishops Mount, Stratford upon Avon
Tel. 0789 298227

British Aikido Federation
29 Abberbury Road, Iffley, Oxford
Tel. 0865 777022

The Alexander Technique
The Society of Teachers of the Alexander Technique
10 London House, 266 Fulham Road, London SW10
Tel. 01-351 0828

ASSET
(The National Association for Health and Exercise Teachers), 202
The Avenue, Kennington, Oxford OX1 5RN
Tel. 0865 736066

Athletics
Amateur Athletic Association
Gen. Sec. M. Farrell, Amateur Athletic Association, Francis House,
Francis Street, London SW1P 1DL
Tel. 01-828 9326

Cycling
British Cycling Federation
Sec. L. A. Unwin, 16 Upper Woburn Place, London WC1H 0QE
Tel. 01-387 9320

Dance

Association of Dance and Mime Artists
9 Fitzroy Square, London W1
Tel. 01-388 9848

The Association for Dance Movement Therapy
99 South Hill Park, London NW3
Tel. 01-769 0924 or 01-834 4533

British Amateur Dancers' Association
Sec. S. Wells, 14 Oxford Street, London W1N 0HL
Tel. 01-636 0851

British Ballet Organisation
39 Lonsdale Road, London SW13
Tel. 01-748 1241

Chantraine Method
Miss Patricia Woodall, Chantraine School of Dance, 47/3 Compayne
Gardens, London NW3 6DB
Tel. 01-624 5881

Chisenhale Dance Space (for Post Modern, Acrobatics, Performance
art)
64–84 Chisenhale Road, London E3
Tel. 01-981 6617

Council for Dance Education & Training
5 Tavistock Place, London WC1H 9SS
Tel. 01-388 5770

Dalcroze Society
Sec. Mrs A. Heron, 89 Highfield Avenue, London NW11 9TU
Tel. 01-455 1268

Dancercise
Phyllis Greene Morgan, The Barge Durban, Lion Wharf, Old
Isleworth, Middlesex
Tel. 01-560 3300 or 568 1751

Dartington College of Arts (for Modern and Post-Modern)
Theatre Dept., Dartington Hall, Totnes, Devon TQ9 6EJ
Tel. 0803 862224

English Folk Dance & Song Society
Sec. Mr Maynard, Cecil Sharp House, 2 Regents Park Road, London
NW1 7AY
Tel. 01-485 2206

Laban Centre for Movement and Dance
University of London Goldsmith's College, New Cross, London SE14
Tel. 01-691 5750/4070

Laban Guild
Sec. Mrs Pocock, Yew Tree Cottage, Hardham, Pulborough, Sussex
RH20 1LB
Tel. 0798 22839

London Contemporary Dance (Contact Improvisation &
Release and all contemporary styles)
The Place, 17 Dukes Road, London WC1
Tel. 01-387 0161

London Contemporary Dance Society
The Place, 16 Flaxham Terrace, London WC1
Tel. 01-387 0324

Margaret Morris Movement
Admin. J. Hastie, Suite 3/4, 39 Hope Street, Glasgow G2 6AG

Medau Society
Sec. Mrs H. Hewitt, 8b Robson House, East Street, Epsom, Surrey,
KT17 1HH
Tel. 78 29056

Moves Fitness
Barbara Dale, Body Workshop, Lambton Squash Club, Lambton
Place, Westbourne Grove, London W11
Tel. 01-221 7989

National Resource Centre of Dance
University of Surrey, Guildford GU2 5XH
Tel. 0483 571281

Royal Academy of Dancing
48 Vicarage Crescent, London SW11 3LT
Tel. 01-223 0091

Women's League of Health & Beauty
Sec. P. Hutton, 18 Charing Cross Road, London WC2
Tel. 01-240 8456

Eutony
c/o Therese van Cawenberghe, 68 Huntingdon Street, London N1
Tel. 01-607 5248

The Feldenkrais Method
18 Kemplay Road, London NW3
Tel. 01-435 8145

Football
Football Association
Sec. E. A. Croker, 16 Lancaster Gate, London W2 3LW
Tel. 01-262 4542

Women's Football Association
Sec. Miss L. Whitehead, 11 Portsea Mews, Portsea Place, London, W2 2BN
Tel. 01-402 9388

The Inner Game
Courses in Sports and Business, Pennyhill Park Country Club, College Ride, Bagshot, Surrey GU19 5ET
Tel. 0276 76400

Jogging
National Jogging Association
Sec. J. Whetton, Newstead Abbey Park, Newstead, Notts.
Tel. 0623 793496

Judo
British Judo Association
Sec. Miss G. Kenneally, 16 Upper Woburn Place, London WC1H 0QH
Tel. 01-387 9340

Keep Fit
Keep Fit Association
Sec. Mrs C. Roper, 16 Upper Woburn Place, London WC1H 0QG
Tel. 01-387 4349

Lawn Tennis
Lawn Tennis Association
Sec. J. James, Barons Court, London W14 9EG
Tel. 01-385 2366

Martial Arts
Martial Arts Commission
Sec. D. Mitchell, Broadway House, 15/16 Deptford Broadway, London SE8 4PE
Tel. 01-691 3433

Pilates Technique
Pilates Studios Limited
113b Golders Green Road, London NW11
Tel. 01-455 4618

Rambling
British Ramblers' Association
Sec. A. Mattingly, 1–5 Wandsworth Road, London SW8 2XX
Tel. 01-582 6878

Skiing
British Ski Federation
Sec. P. A. Allan, 118 Eaton Square, London SW1W 9AF
Tel. 01-235 8227

English Ski Council
Director: D. Francis, 4th Floor, Area Library Building, The Precinct,
Halesowen, West Midlands B63 4AJ
Tel. 021-501 2314

Ski Skills
12 Ranelagh Road, Redhill, Surrey RH1 6BJ
Tel. 0737 67152

Sporting Bodymind
18 Kemplay Road, London NW3
Tel. 01-435 8145

Sports Councils
Council for Sport in Ireland
Floor 11, Hawkins House, Hawkins Street, Dublin 2
Tel. Dublin 714311

The Scottish Sports Council
1 St. Colme Street, Edinburgh EH3 6AA
Tel. 031-225 8411

The Sports Council
16 Upper Woburn Place, London WC1
Tel. 01-388 1277

The Sports Council for Northern Ireland
House of Sport, Upper Malone Road, Belfast BT9 5LA
Tel. 0232 661222

The Sports Council for Wales
The National Sports Centre for Wales, Sophia Gardens, Cardiff CF1
9SW
Tel. 0222 397571

Swimming
Amateur Swimming Association
Sec. H. W. Hassall, Harold Fern House, Derby Square, Loughborough, Leics. LE11 0AL
Tel. 0509 230431

T'ai Chi
British T'ai Chi Chu'uan Association
7 Upper Wimpole Street, London W1M 7D
Tel. 01-935 8444

International T'ai Chi Chu'uan Association
184/192 Drummond Street, London NW1
Tel. 01-387 5381

Volleyball
English Volleyball Association
Director: G. Bulman, 13 Rectory Road, West Bridgford, Notts. NG2 6BE
Tel. 0602 816324

Weight Lifting
British Amateur Weight Lifters Association
Sec. W. Holland, 3 Iffley Turn, Oxford
Tel. 0865 778319

Yoga
British Wheel of Yoga
Sec. Mrs J. Burling, 80 Leckhampton Road, Cheltenham, Glos.
Tel. 0242 24889

Iyengar Yoga Institute
223A Randolph Avenue, London W9 1NL
Tel. 01-624 3080

Index